HOW TO

PRACTISE COMPLEMENTARY MEDICINE PROFESSIONALLY

BY

RICHARD KNIGHT
BRIDGET MAIN
&
JANET ROBINSON

Published by arima publishing

www.arimapublishing.com

Third Edition 2004

First published 1994 by Cross Roads Publications

Copyright © Richard Knight 1994, 1999, 2004

The Authors assert their moral right to be identified as the authors of this work

ISBN 1-84549-004-5

Drawings by Jane Steward-Rivers, Freelance Artist & Illustrator

Printed and bound in the United Kingdom

Typeset in Palatino 12

Distributed by **The Association of Natural Medicine**
19a Collingwood Road, Witham, Essex CM8 2DY
Registered Charity No 1009714

arima publishing
ASK House, Northgate Avenue
Bury St Edmunds, Suffolk IP32 6BB
t: (+44) 01284 700321
www.arimapublishing.com

Contents

SECTION ONE: From Ethics to Seeing Patients

SECTION TWO: Practical issues in establishing your practice

SECTION THREE: From Record Keeping to Touch

SECTION FOUR: From Sensitive Issues to Taking Care of Yourself

Acknowledgements

The authors wish to take this opportunity to thank all Members, supporters and founders of the Association of Natural Medicine, and in particular all those who have served, and are serving on its Governing Council. We also thank those who made contributions to this third edition as well as to the previous two.

Without our students and you who are practitioners, the need for this book would not have arisen. We hope this publication influences the ongoing development of complementary medicine within a climate of the highest of practice standards and professionalism.

Preface

It is a reflection of how rapidly complementary medicine practice has grown that we have the pleasure of introducing you to this, our third edition. The major change to our practice has been the influence of our developing relationship with European colleagues and consequently evolving legislative requirements. Moreover, the increasing influence of 'umbrella' organisations within the UK, representing their respective therapies, is viewed by us as a positive evolution in practice delivery.

This book has been written to assist primarily newly qualified practitioners in establishing their own practice. The writers of this book are equally confident the material discussed will also be of both interest and value to the more experienced practitioner. It brings together legal, professional, ethical and practise issues and is therefore an essential guide and valuable reference book. The Association of Natural Medicine expects all its Members to adhere to the principles and standards detailed in the following, given that the main reason for producing this book is unequivocally the promotion of the highest levels of practice possible.

The fact that complementary medicine in general is now rightly receiving increasing interest from Government and the general public, places upon us all the professional responsibility of ensuring we each fully acknowledge and accept that responsibility. Our patients deserve and should expect no less. Hence, the Association is represented at, and active in, numerous core organisations and forums including the Parliamentary Group for Integrated and Complementary Healthcare.

We must therefore assume full responsibility for evaluating the quality of our work with the maintenance of our individual professional standards clearly of central consideration. Of course, underlying any meaningful evaluation of our own individual practice must be the motivation to continuously enrich and advance our abilities.

R K   Chelmsford, 2004

Introduction

Complementary Medicine is a professional activity. Implicit in its practice are ethical principles which describe the professional responsibility of the practitioner. The primary objective of a code of ethics is to make these implicit principles explicit for the protection of patients.

Complementary medicine like other similar helping professions is a value laden activity. Such values can be seen as symbols of our humanitarianism. It is therefore fundamental that in the education and training of future practitioners we should aim to equip them with the professional values which must guide their work and accountability. Moreover, this is essential if they are to become, and act, as part of a wider professional group. Basically, the values which inform our work reflect 'respect for the individual' and 'the patient's right to self-determination'.

Probably the most useful way of describing these concepts is that people should be treated as ends in themselves, not as means to ends. Whilst every individual possesses particular features, for example, intelligence, social standing, gender or race, these do not constitute his or her value as an end. In short, each individual person has a legitimate claim to be valued equally and therefore we need to respect each individual's autonomy in the pursuit of their own self chosen goals.

So, whilst it may be acceptable to use rational argument to try to get the other person to change his or her mind, say about particular behaviours, it would be inappropriate for the practitioner to attempt to make him or her change their mind by the exercise of power, collusion or manipulation. (Of course, this is not to deny that 'respect for the individual and the right of self-determination' is qualified in certain circumstances. For example, where a person's actions break the law, or where an individual is a danger to others or his or her self.)

The skilled practitioner enhances the value of 'self-determination' by increasing the patient's capacity to evaluate choices through their active participation and consent. Much of the work within complementary medicine practice has internal change as its goal, although such action on behalf of the patient is likely to be initiated through the physical manifestation of a problem or problems.

Such change is not achieved through giving orders but by the active involvement of the patient who in his or her own time comes to accept, on deepening levels, the process of change. For example, the prescribed remedy or the individual acupuncture treatment will further this change or act as a catalyst for change. Needless to say, the task of this book is not to attempt to resolve the philosophical and moral implications faced implicitly by practitioners, but rather to acknowledge that a 'values' perspective plays a critical role in our attempts to understand both professional theory and practice.

In training practitioners it is never sufficient simply to concentrate on the 'techniques' of a given therapeutic intervention, as involvement with the patient is never purely a 'technical transaction' but one that also operates on, and presupposes an acceptance of a set of core professional values.

Therefore the structure of this book commences with an investigation of the broad philosophical and moral questions facing us in practice and then endeavours to answer if not all, many, of the questions requiring answers for those in practice or in the process of establishing a practice to initially consider.

Remembering always the aim of the complementary practitioner is to assist the patient back to full health, strength and well-being at a physical, mental, emotional and vital energy levels, or spirit areas of consciousness. The body of the book responds to a broad range of issues that are inherent within that process.

So that the material can be utilised for easy reference a question and answer style has been adopted.

In order to ensure consistency and avoid any ambiguity the term 'patient' is used throughout the book and should be taken to also equate with such definitions as 'client' or 'helpee'. In addition, the term 'practitioner' is used consistently but can equally represent such descriptions as 'therapist' or 'helper'.

'He/She' is adopted throughout the book so as to avoid any gender bias. In the few occasions where 'He' or 'She' are used singularly gender bias is not intended.

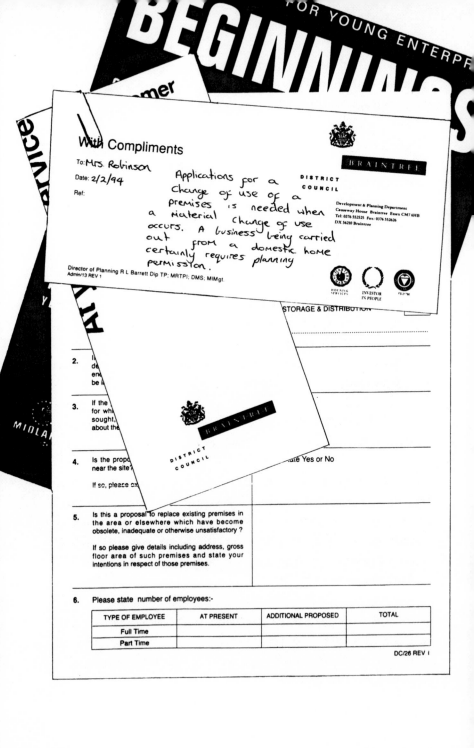

With Compliments

To: Mrs. Robinson

Date: 2/2/94

Ref:

Applications for a change of use of a premises is needed when a material change of use occurs. A business being carried out from a domestic home certainly requires planning permission.

BRAINTREE

DISTRICT COUNCIL

Development & Planning Department
Causeway House Braintree Essex CM7 6HB
Tel: 0376 552525 Fax: 0376 552626
DX 56210 Braintree

Director of Planning R L Barrett Dip TP; MRTPI; DMS; MIMgt.
Admin/13 REV 1

HOUSING SERVICES   INVESTOR IN PEOPLE

BRAINTREE

DISTRICT COUNCIL

STORAGE & DISTRIBUTION

....

2.

3. If the
for wh
sought,
about the

4. Is the propo   ate Yes or No
near the site?

If so, please ex

5. Is this a proposal to replace existing premises in the area or elsewhere which have become obsolete, inadequate or otherwise unsatisfactory?

If so please give details including address, gross floor area of such premises and state your intentions in respect of those premises.

6. Please state number of employees:-

TYPE OF EMPLOYEE	AT PRESENT	ADDITIONAL PROPOSED	TOTAL
Full Time			
Part Time			

DC/26 REV 1

14

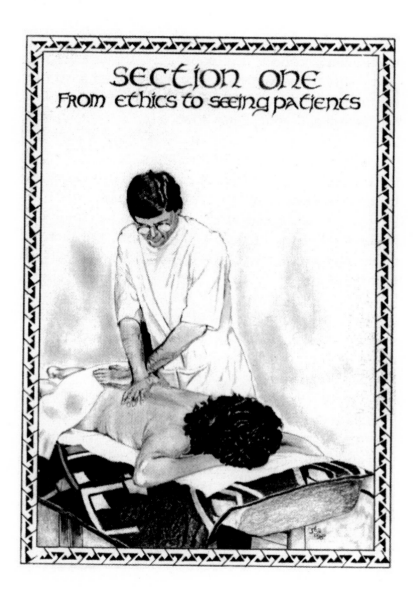

SECTION ONE
FROM ethics to seeing patients

What do we mean by a Code of Ethics?

A code of ethics is about the principles that relate to a practitioner's conduct, responsibility to patients, responsibility to colleagues, responsibility to employer or employing organisation, responsibility to the profession as well as responsibility to society.

The ethical issues that we encounter as practitioners are, quite clearly a sub-set of ethical issues in general, those upon which our laws and values are based. In other words actions which are inherently right or good, or good by virtue of their consequences and thereby emphasise our obligations to others and respect for their rights and protection.

The following standards of ethics are intended to aid practitioners of natural medicine in the maintenance of the highest standard of professional conduct:-

- Practitioners should improve their knowledge and skill on a continuous basis so that they may offer the very best standard of treatment to the patient, and contribute to the improvement and advancement of the therapy.

- Practitioners must consider the patient according to holistic principles. By this we mean looking at the whole person as opposed to specific symptoms only.

- At all times, practitioners should honour the patient's integrity, individuality and privacy, and maintain confidentiality.

- Practitioners should at all times consider the safety and welfare of the client.

- Practitioners must respect the patient's right to be treated as an individual which embraces the notion of personal differences including race, culture, age, gender, intellectual, physical and socio-economic position. In short the recognition that everyone is unique.

- Practitioners must record findings and clinical data methodically and without distortion and take account of the patient's rights to inspect their case record.

- Practitioners should recognise the value of other therapies and work with other practitioners and/or refer patients to them when it is in the patient's best interest.

- Practitioners should in no way exploit the patient. For example, by misusing their authority to dominate patients to the detriment of their well-being, or establishing with the patient a 'relationship' which is outside of the boundaries of their practitioner role, for example, asking a patient to lend them money or to undertake specific tasks for them in a way that could be seen as exploitative.

- No claims must be made by practitioners either verbally or in writing for the cure of any given disease.

- Practitioners who are Members of, or Registered with, the Association of Natural Medicine should be aware that the ethics of this Association must be observed and that by doing so the good name of the Association, and its Register, and the needs of the patient, will be best served.

The Association of Natural Medicine operates a disciplinary procedure and will convene a Disciplinary Committee when ever appropriate. (See *Annex 1* at the end of this book). Failure to observe these ethics will result in the respective practitioner being referred to the Disciplinary Committee and may result in the practitioner's name being removed from the Register.

Moreover, it is the policy of the Association of Natural Medicine to require of all of its students and Registered practitioners to disclose, within the framework of the Rehabilitation of Offenders Act 1974, criminal convictions. (See *Annex 2* at the end of this book).

Practitioners should also be fully insured for professional indemnity and public liability.

Practitioners should not misrepresent themselves in any way regarding their training and qualifications, which may be misconstrued by patients as evidence of having an orthodox medical background. (See *What title can I use?*)

What is the meaning of a 'true professional'?

We know from the work of people like Carl Rogers (1967) and his client-centered approach that the true professional is not someone who is distant, cool and pompous but is someone who shows a warm manner, friendliness, someone who convinces the patient of his active interest in, and concern for, the patient's position. Not appearing bored but listening attentively to what the patient has to say, apologising if you are, for example, interrupted. Paradoxically being a 'friend' rather than a 'professional' but not friendship in the conventional sense.

Being a true professional is also about setting clear boundaries in terms of expectations and obligations. Moreover, it is important to always remember that the practitioner's role places you in a position of power and privilege over your patient. Professional practitioners carry their authority in the knowledge that it is their job to give structure to the helping relationship, to direct and make positive use of verbal exchanges, to always explain what is going on including the potential and indeed limits of any specific therapeutic intervention.

Patients often come with unrealistic expectations of you - 'I understand you can cure me?' - so it is imperative to ensure that an honest and genuine framework is set in terms of what may or may not be achievable, otherwise the relationship will be a deceitful one.

You also have an obligation to never misuse or abuse the 'power' that is invested, by the patient, in you. The majority of patients appreciate and accept the helpers 'superior knowledge'. This position must be held with humility and modesty.

Practitioners wish to see people change and get well but remember practitioners, like their patients, experience stress, grow older, have their own aches and pains, worry about their children and so on.

What principals and guidelines should I use in practice?

- Be clear with the patient how much time is available.

- Ask them why they have come to see you.

- Help the patient to be relaxed and unafraid.

- Try to have empathy with patients - to see and hear things through the patient's eyes and ears.

- Do not be judgmental or condemnatory. Try to show acceptance and tolerance.

- Smile on first acquaintance. This may help a patient to communicate more freely.

- Do not ask questions that can be answered simply yes or no. Open-ended questions are likely to provide more information, for example 'Tell me more', 'Can you explain this issue more fully' and so on.

- Do not 'put answers in the patient's mouth', and allow the patient to speak freely without unwarranted interruption.

- Beware of probing too deeply, too quickly, and it is inappropriate to probe deeply at all unless there is a clear purpose in doing so.

- Do not be afraid of silences when patients are thinking their way forward. Having said that, it is important not to prolong silences, when to do so would be felt uncomfortable. (Jamieson 1978)

What qualities make a good practitioner?

There are almost as many kinds of helpers as there are people who need help. There is probably no one person who is an ideal helping person so that each of us will probably lack some of the qualities a helping person should have. (Knight 1992)

- The enjoyment of being alive: maturing, living, growing, developing.

- The acceptance of change.

- Seeing all people, including oneself, as being involved in problem solving.

- Being creative, intellectually open, receptive.

- Recognising that most problems in life are tentative.

- Self-awareness and genuineness.

- Self-knowledge, self-respect, self-confidence.

- A desire to increase patients' freedom of choice and control over their lives.

- The courage to confront patients with the reality of their problems.

- The courage to risk failure in pursuing clinical objectives.

- The professionalism to cope with the unpredictable and the courage to face the criticism and blame for one's actions.

- Sensitivity to the patient's feelings, doubts and fears. (Compton and Galway 1975)

Are there any kinds of people that do not make good practitioners?

Experience suggests that there are four kinds of people that do not make good practitioners in helping:

- Those who are interested in knowing about people rather than in serving them.

- Those who are impelled by strong personal needs to control, to feel superior, to be liked.

- Those who have resolved problems similar to those experienced by people in need of help but who have forgotten the personal price it cost them to do so.

- Those who are primarily interested in retributive justice and moralising.

The qualities of awareness and sensitivity are the essential prerequisites for a good practitioner.

What things are important to remember when meeting new patients?

Each new patient represents a familiar, even a routine process for the practitioner, while for the patient the occasion is probably unique. Many new patients have described how much determination they needed before they could bring themselves to cross the threshold of the clinic. If, having achieved this, they are greeted with a casual, cavalier or hostile attitude, they are obviously likely to leave then and there and never come back.

Many of your patients will have intensely emotional reasons for visiting you and therefore the need for even more sensitivity and tact is required. Remember it is our daily and life events that reflect the similarity between all of us.

Nevertheless, it is the very inequality in the clinical relationship and our obligations to a patient that are the core factors of professional identity. We must:

- Involve the patient in their own self development as much as possible.

- Make our own objectives explicit.

- Be honest in explaining to the patient how we are assessing their situation.

- Be open about the responsibilities implicit in our role.

Do I need any licences to practise?

If you practise massage, aromatherapy, acupuncture, electric treatment, chiropody, reflexology or other similar treatment you should apply to your Local Authority Trading Standards office to enquire whether you need a licence to practise your particular therapy in your area. Each Council has their own byelaws which vary from one area to another.

In some areas some of the above mentioned therapies may not be considered licensable but you may still need to register with your local District or Borough

Council under the Local Government (Miscellaneous Provisions) Act, 1982.

It should be noted that it is the premises, rather than the individual that is licensed. If you work from your own home, inviting members of the public for treatment then your home must be licensed. If you treat your patient in their own home then a licence is not required.

The application for a licence must be made by the person responsible for conducting the business. Information required is detailed on form 5002, also each person wishing to carry out treatments on the premises must complete form 5003 or 5004, depending on the treatment to be offered. These forms are available from your Council Trading Standards Office. In addition to completion of the forms and their requirements an inspection will be made of the premises.

There is a fee charged for the issue of the licence, which is renewable each year. (See *Are there any regulations regarding practising massage, acupuncture, or other body contact therapies from home*)

As mentioned above, in most areas, you do not need a licence to practise acupuncture. However, you will need to register with the local Council in any area of the country that you are going to practise. (This applies to the UK - in other countries Local and National Laws will apply.) On application to Register, the Council will need to know the particulars of the premises where you will be practising, and if you have had any relevant convictions. The Council may have byelaws regarding cleanliness and hygiene of the premises and person, and the disposal of 'sharps' and other waste matter (paper towels, tissues and so on).

To Register, you should apply to the Environmental Services Department of your District Council. There is a fee charged for Registration. Registration does not have to be renewed unless you move premises, or make major changes to your practice.

(Note: Osteopathy and Chiropractice are now State Registered professions, Herbal Medicine and Acupuncture are seeking the same registration status. The Homeopathic profession is currently working towards a voluntary National single register.)

The Association of Natural Medicine maintains a Register of all its appropriately qualified and insured practitioners and this is updated annually.
(See *Useful Addresses*)

Is it legal for me to supply remedies?

There are no legal restrictions on supplying oral remedies if you are simply passing on unopened containers that you receive from your supplier.

However, if you buy your remedies in bulk and distribute them in small quantities to your various patients then you require a Licence for 'the assembly of medicinal products' from the Medicine and Healthcare Products Regulatory Agency arising out of the Medicines Act 1968. An annual fee is charged for this License. You make an enquiry to the general information desk

for further advice regarding the relevant department for your specific therapy.
(See *Useful Addresses*)

Insurance cover

Is insurance cover needed to practise complementary medicine?

By Law, natural medicine practitioners are not 're-quired' to hold any form of medical malpractice insurance. However cover is required in today's litigation orientated climate to ensure you are adequately protected against incurring potentially heavy financial losses following a medical malpractice suit including but not restricted to legal costs, compensation and so on.

What insurance cover do I require?

You should have an insurance policy which covers both medical malpractice claims as well as general third party claims. As a minimum, the Association of Natural Medicine insurance brokers recommend approximately £1 million of cover. However, due to market conditions, the Association of Natural Medicine feels that all of its Members should insure against claims potentially in excess of this minimum limit of indemnity. Accordingly, the Association instructs its brokers to offer and advise all practitioners individually of the opportunity to increase their insurance cover to the recommended level of one million pounds. Additionally, the brokers must be advised if any of your work is ever carried out other than solely within the United Kingdom as you may **not** be insured to practise abroad.

What should I do if a claim is made against me?

For legal reasons and as a general insurance requirement you should avoid 'advertising' that you hold insurance cover. If a complaint or claim is actually made against you, the insurance brokers must be advised immediately. You should not admit liability or blame to the other party and any correspondence received from them or any third party should be forwarded to the broker immediately. The insurers recommend that you should not even acknowledge such correspondence.

If you are a Member of the Association of Natural Medicine then the Chairman of the Governing Council must also be notified if the claim is associated with malpractice or breach of the Code of Ethics.

How does a patient go about making a claim?

If a complaint is made against you, or a patient indicates that they intend pursuing a claim against you, it is recommended that you invite them to write down their grievance and forward it to the insurance broker where the entire matter will be handled for you. You may also wish to put 'your side of the story' in writing for the broker's information. As regards quantifying any costs or compensation, this would normally be left in the hands of solicitors appointed by your insurers.

What would happen if I did not have any insurance cover?

Firstly you would not be in receipt of the automatic advice available in dealing with the claimant in the initial instance. Such advice may assist in avoiding a claim at all or in mitigating your exposure. Furthermore you would have to meet legal costs yourself. In a recent claim, defence costs alone amounted to £15,000. Lastly, there is the question of any compensation awarded to the injured party which if enforced could result in the loss of your personal assets.

Is there any other insurance relevant to my practice that I should consider?

If you are running your practice from home you should inform the Insurance Company with whom you hold your Household Contents Policy and Buildings Policy to ensure that your policy is still providing you with full cover. If you use your car for business purposes then it must be insured for this category of cover. You may also wish to consider taking out Health Insurance for yourself. As a self employed person you may need assistance to pay your household bills should you become unable to work for any reason. (See *Useful Addresses*)

What should I do if I have any further questions about insurance?

Contact the Association of Natural Medicine insurance brokers. (See *Useful addresses*)

Does the patient always have the right to confidentiality?

It is believed that if a meaningful, therapeutic relationship is to develop, a patient must be able to assume the information shared with his or her practitioner will be kept confidential. It is also commonly believed that it is ethically wrong for a practitioner to disclose information shared in confidence by a patient with third parties. Therefore, not only does a breach of confidence threaten the likelihood that an effective relationship can be sustained between the practitioner and the patient, it is also considered ethically wrong to betray the patient's trust by sharing confidential information with others.

However, the patient's right to confidentiality may conflict with other prima facie responsibilities. For example, a client may inform the practitioner, in confidence, that he intends to physically harm his estranged wife. In this example, the patient's prima facie right to confidentiality conflicts with his estranged wife's prima facie right to basic well-being. The practitioner's actual duty in this case may be to report the planned injury to the police. Thus, while patients generally have a right to confidentiality, there are instances when the rights of other individuals to freedom and basic well-being must take precedence. Such situations place practitioners in a precarious position.

Patients need to believe that information shared with the practitioner will be held in confidence, and practitioners need to believe that it is permissible in extreme circumstances to breach confidentiality.

Practitioners can avoid placing themselves in this precarious position by not leading patients to believe that information shared by them will under no circumstances be disclosed to third parties without their permission. Leaving patients with the impression of total and unequivocal confidentiality can be misleading and cannot be defended on ethical grounds.

What can be defended is a statement to patients that you intend to treat information shared by them as confidential and that under only extreme circumstances, when the freedom and basic well-being of others is seriously threatened, would you even consider disclosing the information to third parties.

It is important for you as a practitioner to develop trust between yourself and your patient, based not on an unrealistic assumption that circumstances will never warrant disclosing confidential information to third parties, but on your patient's faith in your judgement and ability to decide when a disclosure might be necessary.

In the final analysis, it is your responsibility to assess the extent to which not disclosing the information threatens the welfare of others and to act accordingly. For example, the threat of assault from a patient may initially be treated as a clinical issue, which requires attention and therefore emphasises the practitioner's burden of responsibility and judgment in taking responsibility for continued work or disclosure to a third party. However, if the patient were to persist in this threat to the point where it appeared that he would carry it out, the practitioner would be obliged to breach his 'promise' of confidentiality. It is your belief about the relative benefits of disclosure of confidential information that ultimately determines your decisions about revealing this information.

Patients also need to understand that the genuine practitioner is likely to be operating within a support system with colleagues where clinical issues and cases will be discussed. This must be in the confines of the overall therapeutic process, and therefore is also about enhancing the well-being of the patient. (See also *What are the implications when a patient chooses to change therapists within the same therapy? What happens to the patients record if the patient transfers to another practitioner? Can I keep my records on computer?*)

What of our ethical relationship with other practitioners?

Complementary practitioners must be supportive of other health professionals and in doing so maintain patient confidence.

Most of us would prefer to think of our relationship with our colleagues as one where we are like minded professionals united in a common effort to improve our patients' well-being. However, there may be occasions when it is necessary in order to maintain the overall professional and ethical basis to our practice that questionable practices among some practitioners have to be challenged or exposed.

It is apparent that the kinds of dilemmas you may encounter in practice are normally reduced to questions of what is right or wrong and therefore, by definition, raise questions of ethics and your judgement. It is important for all practitioners to recognise that many of their decisions are, at their foundation, ethical ones. They will involve the difficult problems of human suffering and arouse our emotions as well as our intellect. We cannot afford to regard ethical dilemmas in helping as merely intriguing. Their resolution can deeply affect people's lives. An important goal in attending to problems of ethics within the helping professions is to help you become more sensitive to these often profound dilemmas.

Therefore we have the obligation and duty not to harm, injure or cause unnecessary suffering to another. Unfortunately unprofessional and indeed sometimes serious malpractice takes place. Hence the need for an effective disciplinary procedure to protect all of us is necessary. An example of such a procedure is the one adopted by the Association of Natural Medicine. (See *Annex 1*)

What might be the benefit for practitioners of working with other professionals and agencies?

The work of a practitioner rarely exists in a vacuum. The development of good working links with other colleagues and agencies is especially important. The Association of Natural Medicine provides a network to support its practitioners, the sharing of difficulties and indeed successes. Now, more frequently, we see the attachment of complementary medicine practitioners to various medical practices leading to major advantages for the patient in terms of ease of referral.

Liaison with other agencies demands of the practitioner a level of professionalism and adaptability, which quite properly is becoming more and more required of us. Practice skills and 'Know How' must be of the highest possible standard and involve a real commitment to ongoing study and the improvement of standards.

Clinical practice and knowledge will never stand still. Having said that, the advancement of our professional knowledge can never rely exclusively on our developing clinical experience but will also involve attendance at post-qualifying courses and seminars as well as networking with other colleagues and agencies.

When should I refer the patient to another Practitioner?

If the patient's needs are considered by you to be beyond your specialism, knowledge or skill then referral will be the only correct option.

Also you may find and feel you are unable to work with a particular patient due, for example, to a 'clash of personality'.

If you wish to refer the patient for an allopathic diagnosis or tests, you must exercise care in the way you describe your understanding of the presenting symptoms. For example a Reflexologist is qualified to make a diagnosis which might include an assessment stating sensitivity in certain areas, but it may be outside their competence to put an allopathic medical name to the condition.

What kind of problems may arise as a result of working with other professionals?

The most obvious difficulty is that of professional arrogance. Paradoxically, it is only by working closely together that the detriment such attitudes bring to patients, and differing professions, can ultimately be resolved. Even within the areas of practice which one might assume to be sympathetic to the other, problems can arise.

For example, Mrs Jones was recommended to have reflexology treatment and consequently went to a qualified therapist who in addition to being a reflexologist was undergoing training to become a hypnotherapist.

During the relaxation part of the reflexology treatment the therapist used a hypnotherapy relaxation technique. This resulted in the patient becoming emotionally upset. Unbeknown to the reflexologist, Mrs Jones was receiving psychotherapy for a problem that had not been discussed with the reflexologist.

Mrs Jones, psychotherapist consequently advised her not to continue with that particular reflexologist. In the psychotherapist's opinion it was not helpful to Mrs Jones to have more than one 'psychological helper'. Mrs Jones by going to a reflexologist, by implication, expected a reflexology treatment.

A second example reflects further this difficulty -

Mr Brown is having homeopathic treatment from Mr Roy. During Mr Roy's course of treatment Mr Brown decides to have some massage. The masseur he chooses also practices homeopathy and prescribes a remedy for Mr Brown (without knowing which remedies had already been prescribed). When Mr Roy sees Mr Brown for his next appointment, the treatment has been altered by the Masseur's prescription, neither Mr Roy nor Mr Brown know which remedy the masseur prescribed. The whole programme of treatment had been altered by this intervention.

All therapists should therefore discuss treatment before commencing and be clear about the patient's expectations, and should explain clearly to the patient exactly what the treatment will involve and which therapies are to be employed.

Practitioners should be aware of the treatment given by other complementary disciplines or therapies so as to facilitate co-operation between all the professional services that may need to be involved in any given case.

What problems may occur as a result of being a multi-therapist?

One problem in being a multi-therapist is that a patient may come to you expecting a particular treatment, when you may feel that an alternative, or combination of your therapeutic knowledge would be more beneficial to the patient.

If this is the case then you must explain your views to the patient and why you have reached certain decisions - and allow the patient to make the decision as to which therapy they wish you to use for their treatment. You must not be tempted to use a combination of therapies without the patient's knowledge and approval.

(See *What kind of problems may arise as a result of working with other professionals?*)

What are the implications when a patient chooses to change therapists within the same therapy?

It is in the best interests of the client for the new practitioner to know why this decision has been made and also the details of previous treatment.

In order for the contract of confidentiality not to be broken it is suggested that the client obtains details of their treatment and brings these with them at the first consultation. This will also provide the opportunity for the original therapist to discuss with the client their decision to change.

(See also *What happens to the patient's record if the patient transfers to another practitioner?*)

Are there any problems for the practitioner if the patient chooses complementary treatment as an alternative to conventional medicine?

Practitioners must guard against the danger that a patient, without previously consulting their General Practitioner, may come to you for therapy for a known disorder and later be found, too late, to be suffering from a further serious problem.

Because of this, new patients and existing patients who you have not seen for some time must be asked if they have seen their Doctor, and what advice they have received. If they have not seen their Doctor you must advise them to do so. This advice must be recorded in your case-taking notes for your own protection.

It is legal to refuse medical treatment, therefore no patient can be forced to consult a Doctor, or follow their advice.

How does a patient 'choose' alternative treatment?

The practice of complementary medicine takes place wholly as a result of individual choice or self-selection. In other words, patients choose to seek out the respective practitioner of their own free will. This does not discount that more and more General Practitioners are now referring more and more patients to various complementary medicine therapists.

Can the practitioner choose the patient?

The practitioner is always at liberty to choose to take on, or not to take on, a patient, for ethical or practical reasons. For example, ethically the patient may have extreme views or they may be already receiving treatment from another practitioner. Ethically the practitioner can choose not to take on a client.

On occasion, patients present for treatment with conditions that you feel are unlikely to respond. During such times, the practitioner can be torn between good sense and compassion which makes it difficult to turn the patient away. Sometimes the patient will 'rally' to the amazement of medical and complementary practitioners alike.

(See *What role has the practitioner in the final stage of the terminally ill patient's life?*)

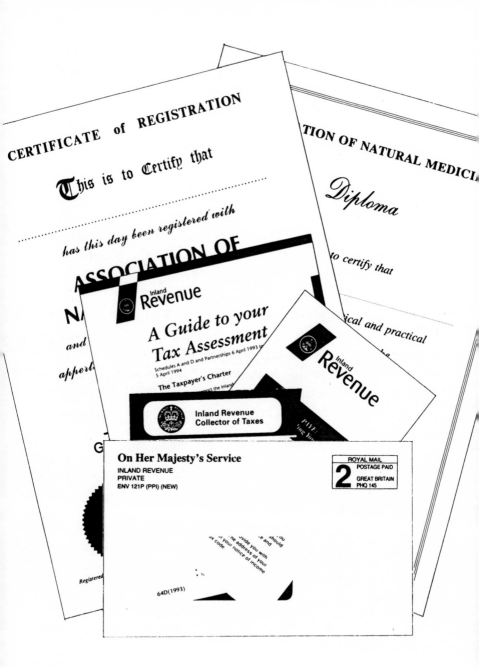

section two
practical issues in establishing your practice~

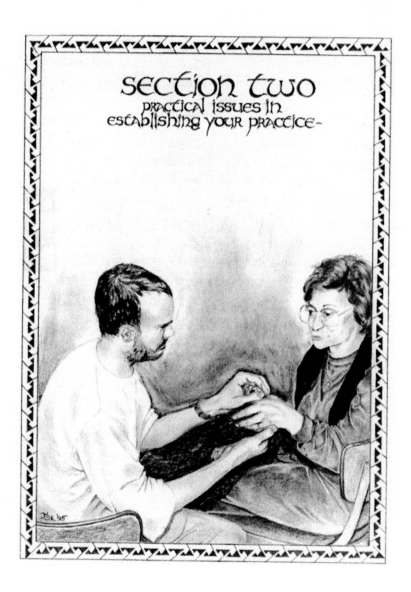

You may advertise a clinic or service but exercise care that nothing is said or implied that would discredit complementary medicine or your profession.

Stationery and name plates should contain minimum information needed to be descriptive but make no claims as to quality or effectiveness of given therapies.

Letters after your name denoting your qualifications and titles can be used. (See *What title can I use?*)

Advertising announcements in the press should contain minimum information necessary as on stationery, and no claims must ever be made about your capacity or ability to cure. You must not make any claims about, or mention treatment of specific diseases.

Standard classified entry in telephone directories should contain name, profession, qualifications, times of surgeries and addresses.

When making public statements, you are advised that you must exercise care and should not present any facts or opinions purporting to represent the views of the Association of Natural Medicine (or similar bodies) without obtaining written consent from the ANM after their examination of the relevant material.

Remember however, advertising is not restricted to 'official statements' in media, but is an ongoing promotion of yourself at all times. Be prepared to talk about the therapy that you offer, both to individuals or groups and societies. Remember to always be polite - and never 'pushy'!

What title can I use?

You should advertise your name followed by the letters of your qualifications, and may give an indication of your therapy, for example Registered Members of the Association of Natural Medicine advertise as follows -

> A B Smith RMANM (Massage)
> C D Brown RMANM (Homeop)
> E F Green RMANM (Acu, Reflexol)

You should not use the title 'Doctor' before your name unless you are a registered physician with the Medical Association in the country of practice.

Complementary practitioners who are not registered physicians but are entitled to use the term 'Doctor' (having acquired the relevant qualifications) may state it after their name with the appropriate qualification, for example -

> Doctor of Acupuncture, China
> Doctor of Acupuncture, Sri Lanka

Practitioners should not refer to their assistant as 'nurse' unless that assistant holds a nursing qualification recognised in the country in which the clinic is being operated.

This whole issue of using 'titles' is about ensuring patients, or potential patients, are not misled into believing you are something you are not, or you hold qualifications which you do not. As noted above, particular clarification is required when and if the term 'Doctor' is being used.

Should I display my certificates?

It is helpful both to the practitioner and the patient to display the Diplomas that are relevant to the treatment you are offering.

You should also ensure that you display your Certificate of Membership from the Association of Natural Medicine (or similar body) in your place of practise.

The Association of Natural Medicine also insists that you display their Code of Ethics along with your Membership Certificate.

You must not display your certificate of Insurance; this is to be produced only in the event of a claim being made against you. The reason for this is that it could be seen as 'an invitation' to make a claim against you.

What do I need to consider when setting up my practice?

To be successful you will need to have a sound idea as to the basis of your practice. Do you intend to establish a part-time or full-time practice? Are you going to develop your own clinic or operate from one already established? What might you require in terms of resources?

Your Local Enterprise Agency is available to help you. Entering self employment requires preparation and planning. There is the paper work, dealing with receipts, knowing how to pay your own National Insurance and Income Tax. Being in business on your own means you are solely responsible for all the decisions as well as debts, and all your personal assets are at the disposal of your creditors should your practice run into difficulties.

It is a fairly simple process to set up on your own as a 'sole trader' and there are no legal formalities assuming you practise under your own name. However if you intend to use any other trading name, your Local Enterprise Agency will provide you with an information sheet on 'Company Names'. If you intend to set up business with a partner or partners, or form a limited company, or set up as a co-operative, then you are strongly advised to consult a solicitor who will draw up the necessary legal documents.

A cash flow forecast is important in order to appreciate the level of finance you need to meet your debts. Your 'cash flow' is the term used to describe the timing of payments into and out of your practice. You can undertake cash flow forecasts reflecting moderate performance, and another showing the optimum situation for you - remembering to estimate all relevant expenses.

If establishing your practice requires more money than you are able to provide yourself then you may need to consider ways of raising the finance. There are numerous methods of obtaining financial loans - overdrafts, term loans, loan guarantee schemes being but three examples. Again, your Local Enterprise Agency will advise you. The most fundamental calculation is for you to be very clear as to what your survival income is to be. That is how much you need each month to pay all personal and business outgoings, for example, mortgage/rent, insurance, housekeeping, electricity, telephone, loan repayments, remedies/oils, stationery and so on. This will highlight the minimum income your practice will need to generate.

Moreover, whatever your kind of practice you need to inform potential patients about the availability of your service - this is your marketing strategy. Remember, potential patients will be looking for, like most 'customers', quality of service at the 'right' price.

You will of course need to identify premises unless, that is, you decide to work from home. How much space you need, the shape as well as the size of your clinic may also be important, access for people with disabilities, toilet and washing facilities, parking and maybe ancillary uses like storage and office space require consideration.

It is advisable to use the services of a solicitor when it comes to conditions of occupancy/renting/leasing of premises. You will need to consider: length of lease, how often rents are reviewed, what are the rates and so on. You should also check with your local Planning Department that you can use the premises for the purpose you intend.

Health and Safety Regulations, Fire Safety Regulations, guidance associated with accidents at work and First Aid facilities may also be something you need to comply with. For further details we advise you to contact your local Environmental Health Service. If you employ anyone you will need Employers Liability Insurance and take account of the recently introduced 'Working Time Regulations' and all associated legislation.

The foregoing is guidance only. For detailed information the relevant authorities in your area should always be consulted. Planning and Licensing requirements vary with the different local authorities. Moreover some deeds forbid premises being used as a business so you may also need to speak to your Building Society.

It can be helpful to discuss your plans with experts such as an Accountant, a Solicitor, a Bank Manager and so on.

(See *Are there any regulations regarding practising from home? Do I need any licenses to practise?, Can you tell me about accounting procedures? and Do I have to register for VAT?*) (See *Useful Addresses*)

Do I have to register for Value Added Tax? (VAT)

This depends on your financial turnover, and the type of business.

You should write to your local Customs and Excise VAT Office for their information leaflet. The address of your local VAT office is in the telephone book under

'Customs and Excise'. The web-site address is www.hmce.gov.uk

You have to Register for VAT if your 'taxable supplies' exceed a specific amount set by Government.

'Taxable supplies' include sale of goods, services provided for payment, supplies made through agents or by self-employed persons.

You can apply for voluntary registration if your turnover is below the required limits, if you feel registration will be of benefit to you. You will have to satisfy Customs and Excise that your activities constitute a business for VAT purposes.

Can you tell me about accounting procedures?

Most complementary practitioners are self employed and therefore for most, the simplest answer is to keep straight forward accounts involving income and expenditure columns, and remember to keep all of your receipts! Then to employ an accountant with experience in small businesses to ensure Inland Revenue and National Insurance contribution requirements are satisfied.

However, it is possible to keep your own accounts and complete the Inland Revenue Self Assessment Income Tax Return.

In all cases you must register as a self employed person, using form CWF 1 from the Contributions Agency, who will then inform the Inland Revenue. You must register with the Inland Revenue within three months - starting from the last day of the month in which your self-employment began. Failure to register within the three months will incur a financial penalty.

You are taxed on your current year's profit and pay in advance (in anticipation of the following year) in two instalments on 31 January and 31 July. Please note that the January payment can also include the residue of any balance of tax remaining payable from the previous year.

How should the clinic be conducted?

You must conduct your clinic to the highest professional standard in your personal appearance, hygiene and decorum, plus hygienic and appropriate decoration, furnishings and so on.

Your premises must be tidy, heated when appropriate and provide washing facilities.

The waiting area should be comfortable and fully insulated for sound from the consulting room.

A nurse or receptionist or assistant should be available when treatment involves the removal of clothes or when you are treating a member of the opposite sex. The actual presence of this third person within the consulting room with you, will be a matter of professional judgement, your knowledge of the particular patient and circumstances, and the need to protect yourself from allegation or attack.

You should not conduct a physical examination of a child under the age of sixteen years except in the presence of a parent or guardian, or other responsible adult known to the child. (See also *What are the confines and appropriateness of touch in the therapeutic relationship?* and *Can I treat children?*)

Case records must be kept secure at all times. (See section on *What hints are helpful on the storage of records*)

If you are offering a dispensing service you must ensure that these items are under supervision when not locked away. Besides protection from theft, the 'mixing up' or 'muddling' of remedies, it is essential also for the proper protection of children.

What about access for people who are disabled?

In order to ensure the Association of Natural Medicine Code of Ethics is met in full and the notion of equal opportunities for all is addressed, access to your clinic must take full account of the particular needs of people who are disabled. Without such provision, large numbers of people would be excluded.

We recognise that alterations and conversions to meet this requirement are not always possible but the Association of Natural Medicine encourages where possible, when adaptations, new buildings and new practices are being undertaken that the issue of access must be part of this process.

Part M of the Building Regulations sets out specifically what is required, for example, ramps, toilet facilities, level thresholds, appropriate door width. It is important to remember that a broad range of disability exists and such factors as induction loops for the hearing impaired and tactile services for people with low vision or telephones at the right height may be other considerations for you.

The best advice can be obtained by contacting your local Access Officer who is usually employed by the District Council. In addition you may choose to contact the Access Committee for England for information and guidance.

In circumstances where such an environment would be impossible to achieve, you may choose to explore the option of referring your patient to a practitioner with premises that are accessible or alternatively consider making a home visit to the patient.

What is involved if I work from home?

Running your clinic from home is an option but there are regulations that are enforced by the Local Authority.

If you, the householder, are the only practitioner working from home then your house remains as a solely domestic building, but only if you use less than ten percent of the total area of the property.

A business being conducted from a domestic home certainly requires a 'change of use' application to the local authority. General nuisance considerations are made, especially regarding parking facilities. The reaction of neighbours is always considered and in residential areas the Council's requirements are usually stringent, although all cases are individually assessed.

Am I vulnerable to more taxes if I work from home?

There is the potential problem of capital gains tax. If you use one room exclusively in your house for business, but charge all or most of the household bills to your business you risk incurring capital gains tax when you sell the property. This means sixty percent of the profit of the house can be taken in tax.

The way to avoid this is to charge a 'management fee' to the business for the use of heating and lighting rather than paying all your bills through the clinic.

Where a room is not used exclusively for business the Inland Revenue would not look to assess you for uniform business rates.

Are there any regulations regarding practising massage, acupuncture, or other body contact therapies from home?

The establishment requirements for license are listed by the Trading Standards Department of your local Council, for example, you may need to have a wash hand basin with hot and cold running water. The current objectives are to ensure the premises used are clean and hygienic, and practitioners have received suitable training. Above all to ensure there is no risk to the health and safety of those people attending licensed establishments.

It should be noted that it is the premises that are licensed and not the individual practitioner. The application form requires details of name, address and two persons willing to give references, and also two passport photographs. A copy of this completed form is sent to the Divisional Police Station. Once all of the references and Police reports (which would include any relevant offences recorded by the police) have been received, and show no objections on which to base a refusal, an inspection of the premises will be conducted by an officer and a report submitted on a standard form. Any licence issued is valid for one year only. At the end of this year a further inspection is carried out and enquiries made whether there are any new employees working on the premises, or if any other changes have been made. (See *Do I need any licences to practise?*)

Are there any regulations associated with practising homeopathy, hypnotherapy, counselling or other non-body contact therapies when practising from home?

Most local Councils set no specific regulations for non-body contact therapies (although it is wise to check in your area as these requirements can vary from one council to another) - the responsibility to ensure patients' welfare and safety remains yours.

How should I organise myself to maximise on the benefits of working from home?

If managed well there will be many benefits in working from home, however when you are new to self employment there may be many distractions.

An area specifically designated for your work is preferable; it is more professional from the patient's point of view to be invited into a room that is obviously your clinic, rather than a corner of your sitting room.

It may also become tiresome re-arranging furniture and the dog each time an appointment occurs, also after this effort it will be extra tiresome if the appointment is missed! It is preferable to set aside a spare room to accommodate your needs, a room which is easily accessible from the entrance. Personal and professional life should be kept separate, and limiting access to your home in this way can help. The room that you allocate should be business like and kept quiet and private during working hours.

The time at which you set your appointments will govern when you work with patients. However time must be allowed for keeping accounts, further study, ordering supplies and so on. Make it a habit to check your supplies - it is unprofessional to rush to the kitchen for oil for your last massage!

Some practitioners may be poorly motivated regarding keeping their books. A set time each week makes this task much easier than a 'scrabble' at the end of the financial year.

To separate 'work' from 'home', a change of clothes may help by making the symbolic statement 'I am now at work'.

The issue of boundaries is also raised with the telephone. When you will be available to answer the telephone for work related matters should be clearly indicated on your appointment card and reinforced at the first consultation. Some practitioners have clearly defined 'phone in' times to ensure their Sunday lunch is not disturbed! If these boundaries are not addressed you may find yourself on twenty four hour call seven days a week.

How important is my appearance?

In the orthodox medical profession it is quite usual for all staff to wear an identifiable uniform. White for Doctors, green for radiographers, blue for nurses, grey for porters and so on. These uniforms provide a link with defined roles within the service.

In the sector of complementary practice there is choice.

Clean white coats certainly look clinical and professional. They obviously provide the necessary protection from oils in touch therapies. For any skin piercing, the white coat also assists in maintaining a clean environment. There is no doubt, a white coat acts as a protective barrier and also adds to the clinical atmosphere. This may also help confirm the intention of the masseuse avoiding misconstrued messages when physical therapy is involved.

In the counselling consultation, a white coat may be interpreted as a barrier. The spoken word and observation are the key tools and the white coat may be seen as stark in this situation.

Professionalism will be maintained by manner, but the clothes you wear should also be considered. Clean, tidy appearance, clothes that you feel comfortable wearing, and that suit your environment are necessary.

You are a professional practitioner and your image should reflect your professionalism.

How do I space my appointments?

Appointments must be spaced to ensure that each patient is given sufficient time. You must be able to 'take the case' without feeling any pressure of time on you, and so that the patient also feels unhurried. Assume your patient may have problems which are complex and allow sufficient time for you to explore the most appropriate options for treatment.

One of the benefits that complementary practitioners offer is that they do 'have time to listen to their patient' rather than the briefer appointment times General Practitioners are able to give.

Patients also generally accept that they may have to wait when they visit their General Practitioner, but they do not expect to be kept waiting when they are paying privately to see a complementary therapist.

Therefore it is always preferable to cater for a 'gap' between patients to allow for the possibility of them being late due to any unforeseen circumstances - rail cancellations, hold-ups on the road, and so on.

If you know that it takes an hour for you to see a patient, then you should consider allowing a few minutes extra before booking your next patient. Taking bookings every hour and a quarter is a useful measure. Or, booking patients for one hour on the understanding that ten minutes of that hour will be for changeover time.

How do I assess my fee for a consultation?

Often practitioners are more concerned with their 'healing' obligations to their patients rather than with the financial aspects of their work. It remains important however, to value the service you offer and avoid demeaning your therapy and your profession by undercharging or overcharging. Each practitioner will find a figure to personally answer this aspect of practice and in doing so will need to refer to the level of service being offered, the expenses of running their practice, the breadth of experience they bring, and the level of fees in their area charged by other practitioners.

Mario Jacoby makes the following interesting comments on this subject:

'The less I charge, the less the patient will feel resentments against me. He will trust me more because he will see I'm not interested in his money but in him as a human being.' These are counter transfer reactions, which often have little to do with the reality of the patient. Behind this can be the unspoken plea 'Please come to me and only stay with me, I am here for you. Let me be helpful, it doesn't cost you much. I need to be your loved companion who tries to help you.'

In other words charging is clearly an issue demanding of you openness, ownership of your decisions with a clear understanding of your patient's own perspective.

An alternative attitude might be -

'I am not ashamed to charge a fee and in that context accept your money. I have worked and studied hard over the past years in order to develop the skill and knowledge to help you. It encourages, and enables me, to know that you have the confidence in me, to then pay my fee, for a 'servant' is worthy of his hire.'

But what about money as a 'symbol' of the specific value of a given treatment?

If the patient has feelings of gratitude or generosity, then money may be used to reflect those feelings. Alternatively a patient may resent the idea of having to feel grateful. This resentment may also be defended by the patient thinking 'This consultation isn't worth much anyway.'

You have to ask yourself 'What is my worth?' and operate, as with all other elements of your practice, with sensitivity and awareness.

It goes without saying that your fees may have to be flexible in order to meet the personal situation and circumstances of your patient and to balance your own financial situation.

What if patients actually cannot afford to pay for my services?

As the availability of complementary therapies on the National Health Service is limited, patients have to refer themselves to private complementary practitioners. However, many will be prevented from making this choice due to financial constraints. Nevertheless individual practitioners have found various ways of adapting to individual circumstances and offering help. Some practitioners offer a sliding scale of fees, where those earning the most also pay the highest hourly rate. This system depends on the honesty of the patient, and of course practitioners cannot easily gauge the patients income status.

Some practitioners request that each patient pay the initial consultation fee in full as a mark of commitment and then negotiate individual arrangements which may even be reduced to covering only the cost of, for example the remedy or oils used.

Some practitioners may be in a position to offer certain clinic times for free treatment. This provides the facility for people to try the therapy and therefore is a useful marketing medium but more importantly provides the opportunity for people to receive treatment who may otherwise not consider doing so.

It must be emphasised that when practitioners offer treatment without payment of a fee, they work under the same professional obligation to the patient as when a fee is paid.

Our aim should always be to empower the patient and support them on the path to health. We do not want to encourage the development of relationships built on a feeling of indebtedness. Such an outcome would be detrimental to individual autonomy and the ultimate aim of the consultation.

What if a patient fails to arrive for an appointment?

If this is the first time the patient has sought help, it may well mean they have simply changed their mind. It can take considerable courage for a patient to make the appointment in the first place and their fear may be overwhelming to the point that they cannot keep the commitment. The practitioner must decide whether to encourage a further appointment by writing or tele-phoning, or whether to accept that person's decision and make no contact. This will of course depend upon the details already known about the patient from the contact made before the appointment.

When the relationship is more developed between the patient and yourself and is based on openness and honesty, appointments will generally be kept. Occa-sionally however, a patient may not arrive. Usually if the relationship is sound, most patients will make con-tact with an explanation for their absence. It is impor-tant to maintain a balance between observing a patient's right to choice, concern for their welfare, and the running of your practice in a business-like manner.

If a client constantly misses appointments with no explanation then you may consider sending an invoice for part, or in some cases even the full fee of the missed appointment. Usually a practitioner will display a notice in the clinic stating there will be a charge for missed appointments.

The following draft letter may also assist you -

Dear ....,

As you are aware your appointment on .... was missed. There may be a simple explanation for this and I would like to give you the opportunity of making a further appointment. Please telephone between .... on weekdays if an appointment is required.

You realise from our previous contact that a fee is payable for appointments missed. I would appreciate settlement in due course.

Thank you.

My kind regards,

Yours sincerely,

What provisions should be made when I am away on holiday?

The helping profession can be extremely demanding and therefore, to ensure your own health and vitality are maintained, regular breaks are required. Your appointment system will obviously allow for this and it is not only courteous, but good practice to inform patients, who may need to contact someone, to have a reliable colleague willing to answer queries and provide support during your absence. It is important, however not to cultivate a sense of your own indispensability.

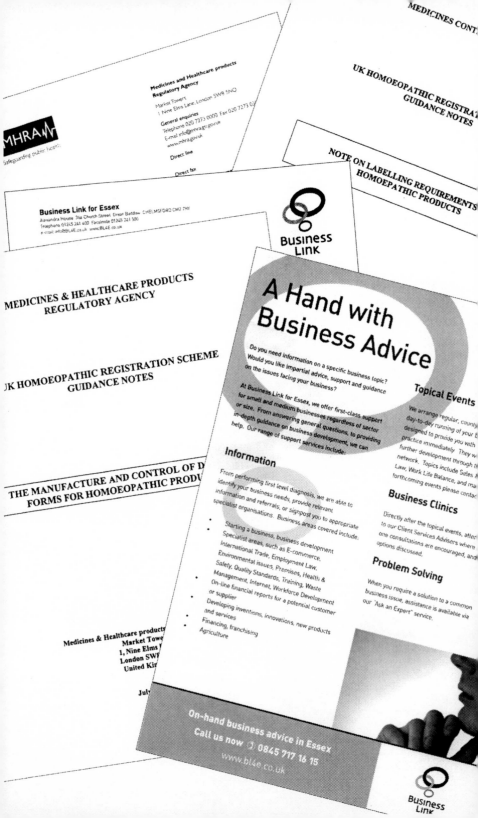

MEDICINES CONT

UK HOMOEOPATHIC REGISTRAT
GUIDANCE NOTES

NOTE ON LABELLING REQUIREMENTS
HOMOEPATHIC PRODUCTS

Medicines and Healthcare products
Regulatory Agency

Market Towers
1 Nine Elms Lane, London SW8 5NQ

General enquiries
Telephone 020 7273 0000 Fax 020 7273 0
E-mail info@mhra.gsi.gov.uk
www.mhra.gov.uk

Direct line

Direct fax

Business Link for Essex
Alexandra House 36a Church Street, Great Baddow CHELMSFORD CM2 7HY
Telephone 01245 241 400 Facsimile 01245 241 500
e-mail info@BL4E.co.uk www.BL4E.co.uk

Business Link

MEDICINES & HEALTHCARE PRODUCTS
REGULATORY AGENCY

UK HOMOEOPATHIC REGISTRATION SCHEME
GUIDANCE NOTES

THE MANUFACTURE AND CONTROL OF D
FORMS FOR HOMOEOPATHIC PRODU

Medicines & Healthcare products
Market Towe
1, Nine Elms
London SW
United Ki

July

A Hand with Business Advice

Do you need information on a specific business topic?
Would you like impartial advice, support and guidance
on the issues facing your business?

At Business Link for Essex, we offer first-class support
for small and medium businesses regardless of sector
or size. From answering general questions, to providing
in-depth guidance on business development, we can
help. Our range of support services include:

Information

From performing first level diagnosis, we are able to
identify your business needs, provide relevant
information and referrals, or signpost you to appropriate
specialist organisations. Business areas covered include:

- Starting a business, business development
  Specialist areas, such as E-commerce,
  International Trade, Employment Law,
  Environmental issues, Premises, Health &
  Safety, Quality Standards, Training, Waste
  Management, Internet, Workforce Development
- On-line financial reports for a potential customer
  or supplier
- Developing inventions, innovations, new products
  and services
- Financing, franchising
  Agriculture

Topical Events

We arrange regular, county
day-to-day running of your E
designed to provide you with
practice immediately. They w
further development through t
network. Topics include Sales &
Law, Work Life Balance, and ma
forthcoming events please contac

Business Clinics

Directly after the topical events, after
to our Client Services Advisers where
one consultations are encouraged, and
options discussed.

Problem Solving

When you require a solution to a common
business issue, assistance is available via
our 'Ask an Expert' service.

On-hand business advice in Essex
Call us now ☎ 0845 717 16 15
www.bl4e.co.uk

Business Link

SECTION THREE
FROM RECORD KEEPING TO TOUCH

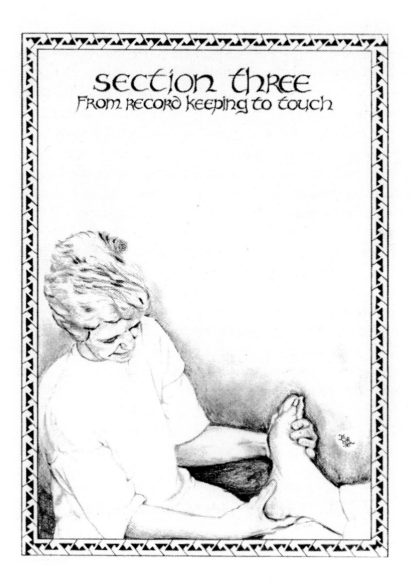

What principles should inform the keeping of case history records?

Patient case history records, apart from being an essential aspect of the patient-practitioner contract, are also legal documents, admissible as evidence in a Court of Law. Since the recent trend from America is for patients to become more litigious, with thousands of dollars being awarded for the 'pain and suffering' associated with practitioner negligence or malpractice, it is more important than ever for all professional practitioners, from all backgrounds to keep accurate, legible and confidential records of the patients whom they see.

These case history records will always need to be produced in the event of any legal action taken on the part of a patient, and it is imperative that a comprehensive and responsibly kept case history is seen to exist. On no account should there by any ambiguous entries, later interpolations, or unexplained alterations to earlier entries, as these raise obvious suspicions as to the validity of the entire document.

Therefore, try to write legibly and concisely, using a minimum of abbreviations, other than those which are universally understood by those in your discipline.

How might I begin to approach this critical task of case history keeping?

Begin by recording the identifying data of each new patient before you take the case. This includes such basic information as full name, date of birth, marital status, address, telephone number, occupation (or previous occupation if retired), height and weight, and the name of their General Practitioner. They may not seem to be a very important point at first, but should the patient (whom you have probably never met before) suddenly for reasons of acute conditions, need to leave your clinic, for example, you may have to refer them directly to casualty, or if they had an epileptic attack, you will need to know who to contact.

Moreover, on extremely rare occasions patients have been known to die during a consultation. You would look extremely foolish and incompetent in a court of law if you had prescribed a treatment for a patient for whom you had no identifying information. Therefore you must be sure you deal responsibly with this aspect of your practice. It can be so easy in your enthusiasm to treat someone who 'comes in off the street' with for example a headache, to forgo the formalities of record taking and to move directly on with the treatment. This is unprofessional and must never happen.

It is a very good idea to have your receptionist, if you have one, take the very basic details of a patient's identity, contact address, telephone number and so on at the time of making the appointment. This information, along with appointment times, can be kept separately on postcard sized index cards.

What other advice on record keeping would be of value?

Never take half a case history and then commence with treatment, in order to make the patient feel they have 'had their money's worth'. Additions made on subsequent appointments are always obvious to the trained eye, and alterations made to earlier entries (unless explained by a footnote signed and dated) invalidate your record. It is better to lose a patient rather than hurry this phase of the helping relationship for the sake of expediency.

You must always sign and date every entry to a patient's case history notes. You should be careful to record patients' comments, (even when they are not improving, or are getting worse), medications, and their visits to other practitioners or specialists. It is important to record any clinical tests performed and their results; whether positive or negative. It is not adequate to disregard a test, which has a negative or inconclusive outcome - this too must be recorded, in order to establish that the test was in fact performed, and a result obtained. On subsequent visits, it may be appropriate to repeat some standard clinical tests at intervals, and to record the results. Again it is not sufficient to write 'BP OK', or 'treatment as before'. Record the quantitative result/dose (eg BP 120/80 or 'gave Nat Mur 200c 2 tablets').

Note also any behavioural inconsistencies or abnormalities, which may later prove indicative of psychological instability, for example, intense agitation. Try to do this discreetly but unambiguously, and if you believe you are dealing with a seriously disturbed patient then consult with colleagues or the patient's General Practitioner.

Should I record any advice given to the patient?

Yes, record all advice and information given to the patient, as this represents an aspect of treatment. Should a patient call on the telephone, record their call on the case history sheet, along with any advice or information dispensed. Record the time, date and nature of the call. Do not offer advice or information to a patient without first reviewing their case history. If necessary, offer to call them back if you require time to check their recorded progress.

On no account allow unqualified staff or students to dispense advice or order remedies by telephone on your behalf. Have them take the patient's number, if you are not immediately available, and assure the patient you will contact them as soon as possible.

What hints are helpful on the storage of records?

Whenever possible, keep patients' records in a filing cabinet, preferably under lock and key. If you work away from home, avoid if possible carrying patient records with you to and from the clinic. A briefcase, or the back seat of a car are not the place to store case-histories, remembering always you are responsible for strictly confidential material. However, index cards with patients' basic identifying data and a record of appointments may be kept separately, say at home, for ease of contact. Such records should however, contain the absolute minimum of information (name, address, telephone numbers, and appointment dates). This is a useful back-up system should your clinic burn down, or become flooded, or perhaps in the unlikely event that both you and your receptionist are ill at the same time and it becomes necessary to cancel patient appointments.

How long do I need to keep patients' records?

It is wise to maintain a current list of patients' records going back to those last seen three years ago. These may be kept close to hand in the clinic. Records of patients seen between three and six years ago are probably best kept in a safe dry and locked storage area such as a trunk or cupboard. Some insurance policies insist on patients records being kept for nine years after the patient was last seen, or for seven years after a child reaches maturity.

When patients' records do become obsolete, they must be shredded or burned by you, or in your presence, and never taken to a recycling centre or thrown in the dustbin.

What happens to the patient's record if the patient transfers to another practitioner?

If you need to refer or transfer a patient to a colleague, and would like that practitioner to see the case history notes, you should obtain the patient's consent. Whenever possible, obtain written permission from the patient, and hand the record personally to the patient. Do not, if avoidable, send case history records by post. If unavoidable, send by recorded delivery. If the patient is unable to collect the records directly from you they may send a representative to collect them with a letter of proxy signed by the patient.

Always place the records in a sealed envelope clearly marked 'Strictly Confidential', and 'for the attention of..........', with your name and address also prominently displayed. This applies to X-rays, test results and other confidential material. Ultimately, these records are the patient's property and you have a responsibility to maintain them and to safeguard them properly, bearing in mind also that the patient has the right to inspect their own record on request.

Finally, please remember that patients' records are just as important as any other area of our work. You need to be just as responsible in this area as you are in other areas of your practice.

Can I keep my records on computer?

Any records, including case history records can be kept on your computer. However, you must ensure that any records you keep comply with the Data Protection Act 1984.

This act states:

'That with few exceptions, if you hold or control personal data on computer, you must register with the Data Protection Registrar.'

'**Data users**', who should register but do not, are committing a criminal offence and may be prosecuted.

'**Data users**' are those who control the contents and use of a collection of 'personal data'. This can be any type of company or organisation, large or small, within the public or private sector. A data user can also be a sole trader, partnership, or individual. A data user may not necessarily own a computer.

'**Personal data**' is information about living, identifiable individuals. This need not be particularly sensitive information, and can be as little as a name and address.

If you do keep your records on a computer you may also consider it advisable to keep a 'hard copy' of case histories.

For further information on the Data Protection Act, apply to the Data Protection Office.

Confidential information should only be sent by e-mail when it has had the security of a password attached. Remember, that all the laws governing copyright, Data Protection, defamation, discrimination and other forms of written communication also apply to e-mails. (See *Useful Addresses*)

In the event of my death, retirement or sale of practice what arrangements concerning patient records should be made?

You should, as with your own personal property, make arrangements for the correct disposal of case records in the event of your death.

If you sell or otherwise transfer your interest in a practice you must inform all of your patients of the change and give the name of the practitioner who has taken over.

No information on a patient should be provided to the incoming practitioner without the permission of the patient.

What are the confines and appropriateness of touch in the therapeutic relationship?

It is important for the patient to feel at ease. For some complementary therapies such as massage, aromatherapy or reflexology touch is an integral part of the treatment. The client will expect to be touched and thus be prepared for this interaction - bearing in mind that for some this may be a very new and unfamiliar experience.

The issue of touching patients provokes varied reactions especially among practitioners. Touching provides considerable sensory information to both practitioner and patient regarding one another's feelings, for example, anxiety, tension fear and ambivalence.

Next, and perhaps most important, touching is normal for most people. If you never touch a patient in a greeting and friendly way, the patient may see you as a cold, withholding person. Moreover touching is especially important for a patient who may have had an unrewarding history of either being touched harshly, or not being touched at all. Therefore touching a patient certainly may stir up feelings and thoughts, especially if you the practitioner have problems touching people and this is then conveyed to the patient. Therefore not to touch may avoid problems, but it may also be artificial and limit your ability to help the patient to work through particular issues.

Being close to others, and feeling OK about one's body is an essential element in becoming a 'whole' human being and feeling secure and trusting with bodywork is necessary for effective helping.

Furthermore in the helping relationship you will often be deemed to be a 'parent figure'. Good 'parents' get their needs met from people other than their 'children' (patients). This includes nurturing, closeness, love and approval. When you are with your patient you are not there to 'get' but to give what is needed - caring, acceptance and approval, treatment, remedies, information and so on. Remember the good 'parent' (practitioner) is always aiming to promote the patient's growth and personal autonomy.

A useful guideline for touching your client is that it is OK and highly positive if it will facilitate the accomplishment of the aims of the specific helping relationship contracted between you both, and in doing so avoids creating further problems which the patient does not wish to discuss or solve. There has to be a real sense of OKness on both sides for positive outcomes to arise. (Autton)

Again, this discussion brings into the foreground the need for supervision and peer support. The issues are extensive and complicated and involve very careful judgements. Let us consider other opinions on this matter.

In his early work, Sigmund Freud was impressed by the power of touch in assessing patients who were distraught.

'When I asked the question 'What is the origin of your symptoms?' and received the answer 'I don't know' I took the patients hand between my hands and said, 'You will think of it under the pressure of my hands - at the moment I relax my pressure something will come into your head. Catch hold of it' I was surprised to find that it yielded the precise results which I needed.'

However, Freud later rejected physical contact believing it 'complicated' the helping relationship.

Wolberg (1954) & Menniger (1958), for example, absolutely forbade any touch with clients for fear that it might arouse sexual feelings or bring forth bursts of anger. Wolberg states that 'It goes without saying that physical contact with patients is absolutely taboo!'

Perhaps the most significant use for physical touch in helping relationships is its potential to encourage self-disclosure. After clinical study Patterson (1973) found that patients who were touched enjoyed more self exploration than did clients who were not touched. Touch in this context was defined as ranging between simple hand contact to full embrace.

Older (1982) states 'When practitioners wish one particular theme or message to be emphasised during an interview' he observed 'a light touch can get the therapist's words in capital letters, can announce that this is more important than what has been said before. The touch acts as penetrating oil for the communication'.

Farrah (1971) argues that physical touch can be a most effective channel of non-verbal communication but it has to be 'appropriately timed, in the appropriate context, with the appropriate individual'.

Carl Rogers (1961) found 'Gradually I observed that I was more effective if I could create a physical climate in which the client could explore, analyse understand and try solutions for himself ... I have been forced to recognise that the most important ingredient in creating this climate is that it should be real'.

Within the helping relationship, a sense of personal space is also essential and must be respected, again emphasising the complexity of judgement practitioners need to make and issues they need to be aware of.

How should I react if a patient wishes to touch me?

It must be recognised that some people are much more 'tactile' than others are and this must be born in mind. If it is a patient's nature to touch the person they are talking to - for example your arm, or your knee, depending on your seating arrangement and proximity - to emphasise a point they are making, then it may be offensive to the patient if you appear to withdraw from them.

Likewise if a patient is showing his or her gratitude or thanks to you for the treatment they have received by touching you - or even perhaps kissing you on the cheek, again it could be upsetting for the patient to feel their affection rebuffed by a cool response from you. However, you must remain professional and not get into a return 'clinch'!

However, if you believe the patient's motivation for touching you is of an amorous intent you must ensure that your relationship is clearly defined to be of a professional nature only. You can achieve this by remaining slightly 'distant' from your patient - physically by sitting behind your desk, and psychologically by only using the patients title, Mr/Mrs Smith and not using forenames, and by keeping the conversation strictly relevant to the patient's treatment. Also by ensuring that nothing you do or say can be misinterpreted. Ensure that your appearance and dress are professional and modest, and cannot be misconstrued as inviting or provocative.

If you are offering a 'hands on' treatment such as massage or aromatherapy you may wish to have your receptionist/assistant present throughout the treatment session. Alternatively you may wish to ask yourself if it would be more appropriate to refer this particular patient to a colleague where this type of problem would simply not occur. The essential criterion is the one of maintaining professional boundaries.
(See *How important is my appearance?*)

Some patients may behave improperly - how will I handle this?

This can occur in all therapies, however masseurs and aromatherapists are more likely to confront patients seeking, if not overtly, subtly, some form of sexual stimulation or reward.

As a practitioner you must be prepared for this and take every step to avoid and confront any advance, innuendo, suggestive behaviour, or flirtation. Again ensure you are not alone (especially in your, or the patient's, home) and be very clear about what your therapy is, its benefits, and how you conduct your practice. A firm, decisive reaction is required with a ready statement at your disposal - for example 'I am a professional therapeutic masseur, I do not give other kinds of treatment, if these are required then you should seek a different kind of establishment'. Any ambiguity must be avoided and therefore very clear statements are essential.

The reaction and response of the patient (and your own) will determine whether you decide to continue.

Discussion and support from colleagues will also be helpful.

(See *How should I react if a patient wishes to touch me?* and *How should the clinic be conducted?*)

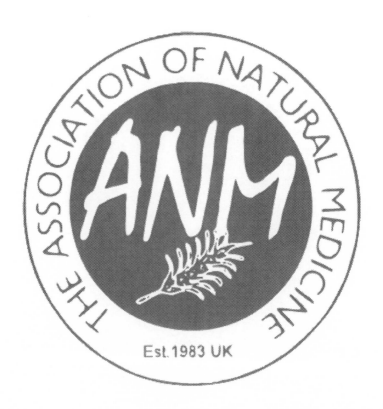

SECTION FOUR
FROM SENSITIVE ISSUES TO TAKING CARE OF YOURSELF

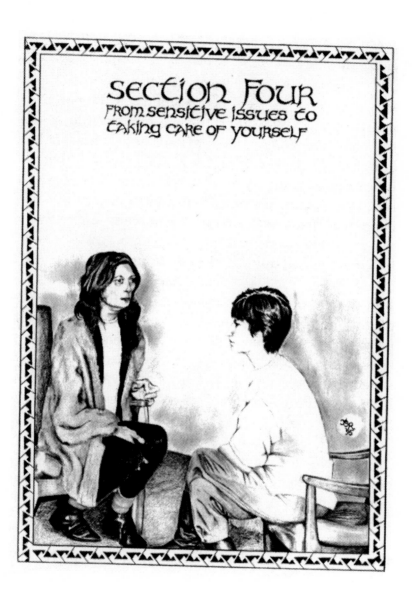

Can I treat children?

Complementary practitioners are legally able to treat children.

However, it is the legal responsibility of the parent or guardian of a child under the age of sixteen to ensure the child has correct medical aid, and indeed it is a criminal offence not to do so. Complementary therapy is not legally approved of as medical aid. Therefore you as a complementary practitioner must ensure that the child has seen his General Practitioner, alternatively you must inform the parent/guardian of this necessity, and must record this statement in your notes.

If the parent or guardian refuses to take the child to the doctor then you must have a signed statement from them saying that they have been informed of their responsibility and asked by you to see their Doctor. This statement would protect you from being named as aiding and abetting an offence should any prosecution occur.

You should not conduct a physical examination of a child under the age of sixteen years except in the presence of a parent or guardian, or other responsible adult known to the child.

What steps should I take if I suspect a child patient is suffering abuse?

This is a highly sensitive area. Your responsibility is to the protection of the child and not the 'protection' of the parent, guardian or adult allegedly involved. If your judgement confirms your belief that the child is being abused then you should discuss the matter with officers from your local Social Services Department (to become, under new Legislation, Children's Trusts. Local Safeguarding Children Boards are to be created as the statutory successors to Area Child Protection Committees). It is the Social Services Department/ Children's Trust which has the responsibility to investigate and have procedures agreed with other relevant agencies, for example the Police, detailing how referrals are to be progressed.

Are there any patients or problems that I should not treat?

Complementary practitioners are forbidden by law to treat venereal disease. This includes Gonorrhoea, Syphilis and Soft Chancre. If you are aware, or suspect, that the patient is suffering from any of these diseases you must refuse to treat him or her for that disease, and must refer him or her to their General Practitioner.

AIDS is not included in the above restrictions and the treatment of it is the individual practitioner's decision.

You must not treat without medical supervision a patient who is in childbirth or for ten days after the birth unless you are also a qualified midwife.

Complementary practitioners are also forbidden by law to treat cancer or to treat TB. Practitioners may support cancer only with the direct permission of a medical doctor. There is indeed a penalty not exceeding two years imprisonment for anyone found to be treating cancer, or for even advising on veneral disease. Our legal adviser states that it is imprudent even to support cancer without the knowledge of the General Practitioner.

Any practitioner offering relaxation therapy / hypnotherapy must abide by the above procedures when dealing with clients suffering from such diseases.
Hynotherapists and counsellors must always check out the psychiatric history of a client during assessment. If a client has a psychiatric disorder then it is advisable not to proceed with treatment.

It is always advisable to seek advice and if in doubt to seek permission from the GP.

List of conditions you are unable to claim cure for:

Diabetes	Bright's Disease
Glaucoma	Cataracts
Epilepsy, or fits	Locomotor ataxia
Paralysis	Tuberculosis

You must not give any dental treatment or advice unless you are also a qualified dentist.

You must not treat animals. (See *Can I treat animals?*)

You must not treat a child under the age of sixteen without first ensuring that the parents know it is their responsibility for the child also to see a General Practitioner. (See *Can I treat children?*)

What should I do about notifiable diseases?

Practitioners must be aware of those diseases, which are notifiable in their country of practice and take appropriate action to conform to the requirements of the local Health Authorities or Laws (see the Public Health (Control of Disease) Act 1984). The person responsible for notifying the Medical Officer of Health is the General Practitioner in charge of the case. If therefore you discover, or suspect, a notifiable disease you should insist that a doctor be called in. Each Local Authority decides which diseases shall be notifiable in its area. There may be local variations but it is assumed that the following diseases are notifiable -

As defined in Section 10 of the Public Health (Control of Disease) Act 1984:

> Cholera
> Plague
> Relapsing Fever
> Smallpox
> Typhus

As defined in Section 11 of the Public Health (Control of Disease) Act 1984:

Food poisoning

As defined in the Public Health (Infectious Disease) Regulations 1988:

Acute encephalitis	Opthalmia neonatorum
Acute poliomyelitis	Paratyphoid Fever
Anthrax	Rubella
Diphtheria	Scarlet Fever
Dysentery (amoebic or bacillary)	
Leprosy	Tetanus
Leptospirosis	Tuberculosis
Malaria	Typhoid Fever
Measles	Viral haemorrhagic fever
Meningitis	Viral hepatitis
Meningococcal septicaemia (without meningitis)	Yellow fever
Mumps	

Where you suspect a patient has signs and symptoms of one of the above notifiable diseases or food poisoning, you should act responsibly by taking the following action:

Advise and encourage your patient to seek a diagnosis from their own GP, and make a record of this advice on their notes.

Contact your local Environmental Health Officer for further advice and record this in your patient's notes.

Can I work in hospitals?

Practitioners who are not registered physicians or nurses may be invited into hospital wards to practise. Such practitioners must at all times present the highest standards of professionalism discretely and considerately, and also take great care to consult staff in charge. Any action, or behaviour, or advice giving that could obstruct or conflict with the work of other health professionals must be avoided at all times.

Complementary practitioners should not wear the same white coats as the hospital staff so as to avoid any confusion, but must be dressed appropriately.

The medical practitioner in charge will retain overall charge of the patient's case and will give permission for the treatment to be delegated to the complementary practitioner.

If the practitioner is also a qualified nurse, he/she must act within the Ethics of the Nursing standards, and must also act only under the guidance of the ward management, observing any code of conduct relevant to the hospital and/or the Area Health Authority/Trust.

Can I treat animals?

It is an offence in Law for any person other than a Registered Veterinary Surgeon, or Veterinary Practitioner, to practise, or be prepared to practise, veterinary surgery.

The Veterinary Surgeons Act of Parliament 1966 defines veterinary surgery as:

'The art and science of veterinary surgery and medicine' and states that this shall include: the diagnosis of disease in, and injuries to, animals, including tests performed on animals for diagnostic purposes; the giving of advice based on such diagnosis; the medical treatment of animals; the performance of surgical operations on animals.'

Practitioners must not give any advice, which would be contrary to the diagnosis of a Veterinary Surgeon.

A veterinary surgeon can refer an animal to you for treatment but this **must** be under his/her direct supervision and you are strongly advised to ensure that any such arrangement is appropriately documented in writing.

Giving first aid in an emergency to animals for the purpose of saving life or relieving pain is permissible.

What makes an emergency must be decided by the individual practitioner, if there is any doubt, the advice of the Royal College of Veterinary Surgeons must be sought.

What role has the practitioner in the final stage of the terminally ill patient's life?

This will largely depend on the relationship between you and your patient. However when there is rapport, even if the relationship is relatively new, there can be a place for you.

The patient and family involved must be given an opportunity to decide whether you are 'welcome' or not. As in all good helping relationships, clear communication is essential and a simple statement such as ' You know that it is up to you to decide if you feel I can provide you support. I suggest you may wish to think about this and I will contact you soon' will help to clarify the situation.

The patient and family will have had time during the illness for thoughtful reflection on bereavement and loss and will have been absorbed in the progress and changes in the condition and hoping no doubt that these will change for the better ... maybe knowing in their heart this is unlikely, or feeling indeed that death itself will be a release.

If you are welcome there will be certain expectations of you, depending on the therapy practised. The client may ask for extra pain relief, and it is suggested, that if, in the best interests of the client, you decide to prescribe, for example homeopathic medicines or acupuncture, you must explain with clarity which remedy/points you are using and why, and what relief may be obtained. Leave labelled packets/bottles available so there is absolutely no doubt about your prescription.

There is a legal point worth noting here that a Post Mortem has to be carried out before a Death Certificate can be issued if the deceased person has not been seen by a Doctor in the last four weeks before their death. It is therefore suggested that you ensure the patient sees their Doctor at least on a monthly basis to avoid such an event.

The most frequently asked question is 'Why is this happening to me?' Many practitioners have a firm belief system or philosophy of their own and it can be tempting to attempt to offer an explanation according to their own beliefs. This is rarely appropriate for the patient or family members.

The atmosphere at these times will affect everyone present in a variety of ways. Some will express their anxiety of impending loss in anger and some of this could be directed at you the practitioner. Also you may find it a struggle to remain professionally detached during this time. Your personal feelings may indeed contribute to what is already an emotional situation. If this is so it may be constructive and indeed appropriate for you to withdraw for a time.

You must ensure that you separate your own sense of loss from that of the family. It may be appropriate to state your own feelings: in fact it may be comforting to others. However, you must not place extra burdens on those already distressed by addressing your own personal agenda. Some may even interpret your distress or concern as an indication of guilt on your part. Emotional expression may be, or may elicit, displacement reactions from the client or family, guilt associated with the situation is perhaps easier to cope with if this guilt is focused on you the therapist!

The role of the practitioner is primarily with the patient. The role is one of providing a listening and hearing ear for comfort and support.

Your discreet withdrawal and focused sensitivity for the patient's privacy will also need to be rigorously observed.

Your future relationship with the bereaved will warrant clarification. They may find it helpful to retain contact or to utilise your skills in a more formal way.

How might I help the bereaved?

Bereaved people need to be reassured that they are not going 'mad', and what they are experiencing is normal, even though it is very painful. Remember that the majority of people die in hospital but most of the grieving will take place at home. The time of bereavement is a crisis in the person's life but it can be a time of personal growth as a new but different life is found.

You must be aware of your own emotional responses when dealing with dying and death, and use your skills of communication and understanding to provide the highest possible level of support.

You will make time to:

- Listen and be sensitive to the bereaved person's feelings and inner needs.

- Facilitate discussion of anxieties, fears and suspicions regarding possible guilt and irrational fears.

- Be as optimistic as the situation permits to avoid any sense of hopelessness.

- Explain and offer support in the process of bereavement and grieving.

Grieving is a natural process through which many people progress using their own resources, and usually with the help and support of family and friends.

During the state of numbness and disbelief, which may happen immediately after the death and last for several hours or days, it may be necessary to prompt the bereaved relative to talk about their loved one in order to start the process of grieving. Often the newly bereaved person feels the urge to cry out, to search and try to find the person who has died. There may be anger and irritability with the practitioner. Intense feelings of guilt may arise - 'I could have done more for him'. A period of apathy and depression may follow.

The most useful thing you can do is sit and listen. There is usually an outpouring of emotions and feelings.

Hasty decisions can be made during bereavement, for example, moving house. This can be disastrous and serve only to prolong the grieving process. The bereaved person should be invited to reconsider major decisions and wait until their lives become more settled. Clearly, absence of grief - in situations when it would normally be expected - should be taken as a sign that all is not going as it should. In such a situation the practitioner will invite the bereaved person to consider more fully his feelings and if necessary refer to a more skilled clinician.

Normal bereavement involves a sense of numbness, which can last for a few days. At this time shock and disbelief act as a defence as the bereaved person tries to deal with the reality of death. There may be episodes of severe distress and at other times little sign of outward emotion. However, as the reality of the loss begins to be absorbed, the grief becomes more prominent. As the feelings of numbness fade, the pain of grieving increases. There may be a need to search for the dead person and this searching, accompanied by crying, is seen as pining and preoccupation with thoughts of the dead person. However, as the searching continues without result, feelings of helplessness and anxiety may increase. Anger is often expressed at the dead person or you the practitioner. Anger may also be shown towards 'God' and the bereaved often go over and over the events surrounding the death trying to make sense of what has happened.

Guilt may be felt, especially if there has been disharmony before the death, for example, for the wife whose husband leaves home to go to work following a row and suddenly dies. Moreover, if it has been an ambivalent relationship, guilt may be pronounced. Many unresolved conflicts may exist, even an unexpressed death wish which has now come to fruition. As grief deepens, anxiety increases and associated physical sensations like tightness in the chest and breathlessness may follow. Agitation and restlessness are common in an attempt to reduce and cope with the feelings of grief. Many varying stimuli act as triggers for grief, such as hearing a favourite tune or meeting with a sympathetic friend.

With time there is a gradual lessening of the feelings of acute grief although feelings of despair and depression may follow. The bereaved may become socially isolated as they may become uninterested in everything around them. This may continue for many months until there is a gradual acceptance of the loss and new roles. A new identity is developed, as roles which were those of the dead person are taken on and self-esteem is strengthened.

These stages are not clear cut and there is no straightforward progression from one to another. Pangs of grief may be felt for many months or years after the death - perhaps as a memory is stimulated. However, with time most bereaved people are able to live again, although altered by the experience of loss.

It is clear that the role of the practitioner is obvious and his skills of listening, attending and being with the bereaved person can make a significant contribution through the process of bereavement and grief and the 'recovery' which follows.

What guidance is helpful in assisting the practitioner to adopt an informed approach to suicide?

One thing that is guaranteed to shock most of us is to hear that someone close to us (and this person may in fact be a patient) has committed suicide. It is not unusual for certain patients to say 'I am going to kill myself'. You are not responsible for the patient's behaviour - we each own our own behaviour. Your role is to ensure your response is both appropriate and informed and that others are notified accordingly if you judge this to be necessary. It is worth being aware of at least some of the facts. Two types of suicidal acts may be distinguished:

1   A serious intent to produce death where careful plans are made and in such cases attempts to commit suicide are often successful.

2   Suicidal gestures (known as para-suicide) involving for example, overdoses or self-mutilation occur but do not usually produce death.   (This is not to assume there is a clear dividing line between the serious intent and the accident.) Parasuicide is more than ten times as common as the first and successful suicide is commoner in men than in women.   This is in contrast to parasuicide, which is commoner in women.

The range of facts known about self-intentioned death assists us in appreciating how complex this issue is:

- The commonest method of self-intentioned death is self poisoning: the overdose.

- Three times as many men kill themselves as women.

- Three times as many women as men attempt to kill themselves but do not die.

- Suicide is found in both the old and the young - even below ten years of age.

- Suicide is found almost equally at all social and economic levels.

- No other form of death leaves friends and relatives with such long lasting feelings of distress and general disturbance.

A range of theories exist about suicide. For example, aggression turned inwards, retaliation by inducing guilt in others, efforts to make amends for perceived past wrongs, efforts to rid oneself of unacceptable feelings or escape from stress, and the desire to join a dead loved one.

Our current understanding of the theories or explanations remain questionable but it is possible to comment on a number of prevalent misconceptions and myths about suicide:

- **'People who discuss suicide will not commit suicide'** - the fact is that up to three-quarters of those who take their lives have communicated the intent beforehand.

- **'People commit suicide without warning'** - the falseness of this belief is indicated by the preceding statement. There seem to be many warnings, such as the person saying 'The world would be better off without me' etc.etc.

- **'It is only people of a certain class that commit suicide'** - suicide is neither a blight of the poor or a curse on the rich. People in all classes commit suicide.

- **'It is easy to establish the motives for suicide'** - the truth is that there is only the poorest understanding of why people commit suicide and why individuals differ in their reactions to seemingly similar sets of social conditions.

- **'Most of the people that commit suicide are depressed'** - this myth does not account for the tragic fact that signs of the impending suicide are often overlooked in people who are not depressed. (This is not to discount that the majority of depressed people do not at some time think of or attempt suicide).

- **'People who commit suicide must be insane'** - although many suicidal persons may be unhappy most do appear to be completely rational and in touch with reality.

- **'The tendency to commit suicide is inherited'** - there is no evidence to support this.

- **'Suicide in some people is caused by the weather or the moon'** - there is no evidence to support such a belief.

- **'People who commit suicide clearly want to die'** - most people who commit suicide appear to be ambivalent about their own deaths.

Again, you have to make a professional judgement as to the strength or veracity of a patient's claim of intending to commit suicide. You may need to consult with their General Practitioner or family; involve other professionals, for example a counsellor; explore other support systems in the community, for example MIND or the Samaritans.

How should I respond to failures in treatment?

You will have 'failures' - these are inevitable. No system of helping has universal validity or absolute success. It is likely that the study of failures could help you improve your methods more meaningfully than just examining your success! So, what is to be 'done' about failures? (See also *How can I evaluate my work?*)

- Firstly, you may need to go back and question the initial assessment. For example, a person may be contracted to 'deal with aggressive feelings more appropriately' but really need to be working on 'getting close to people'. The patient's resistance to change could be the result of failure to identify what he or she really needed.

- Another problem may have to do with the patient's projection of issues. That is, the patient generalising his world views or scripts decision into the helping relationship. For example, the over-complying patient who always may have been scripted to always 'be nice to people' and deny his own needs - consequently he is pleasant to the practitioner but fails to improve emotionally or work on his problems ... saying one thing to you but going away doing something quite different.

- Again, people are sometimes slow to change because change means 'giving up' familiar and certain forms of behaviour. They really know that something is wrong with their lives but may go on defending in the belief that defending is equal to functioning. 'For example, justifying a preference for chocolate or cream cakes! Change will not result until the patient also realises that change is possible. Inevitably there are occasions when this stage will never be reached.

Change means meeting crises or problems in new ways. Becoming does not mean becoming free of pain or distress. It means learning to face such realities differently, to change the way we interact with others and most important, to tolerate anxiety or uncertainty.

The process of change is frightening - but often the greatest fear is change itself. New behaviour is unknown, threatening and risky. New strains must be handled, endured, and coped with in the process of growth - there is always the danger of some regression or giving up.

Patients may meet old situations in which their hostility will again flare up and find themselves in their old reaction pattern. This is why continuing support may need to be built into any subsequent contract.

It must be remembered that the two major components underpinning the helping process argued for here are that patients know cognitively and/or viscerally what they need to do to get 'well' and that they can take responsibility for functioning differently. For example, taking responsibility for their aching hips by going to the acupuncturist!

What should I do if I feel I can do no more for a patient and believe it necessary to terminate my work with them?

Many patients who consult a complementary practitioner do so as a last option, often having tried many other, often suppressive, approaches. Although you will always want to do your best, it is not a failure to accept you can no longer offer any further practical help. It would be totally unprofessional and a deception to continue to offer treatment, knowing there will be no positive benefit.

However, the question of termination of helping is often a difficult one to answer. No patient reaches perfection and there will always be issues to work on and ways in which to improve. At some stage, however, the helping relationship reaches a point of diminishing returns - the time, energy and possibly money, spent in helping outweighs the benefits which a given patient is receiving.

The final decision about concluding your helping will involve you the practitioner and patient. Your responsibility is to give feedback regarding how you see the patient with regard to the goals of treatment. Has the patient met the goals, if not why, and is terminating helping a way you, or the patient, are using to avoid the agreement between you?

When reaching this decision, there is an important balance to observe. Examine your relationship with the patient and ask yourself what you think they expect - ask them also! Value the benefit to them of the 'counselling' side of the therapy. You will need to hear from the patient how he/she is feeling and thinking about ending treatment with you:

- Does this termination make sense to him/her?

- Does he/she feel satisfied with his/her present way of taking care of him/her self?

- Is he/she providing for him/her self adequate nurturing, and protection, for continued improvement?

At other times, the end of the treatment will be initiated directly by you. When this occurs, the reason should be very clear. It may be that the patient is so involved with his own destructive behaviour that this interferes very significantly with the helping process. This can completely obstruct any opportunity for progress. These are difficult decisions. You must be honest with yourself - there will always be people with whom, for various reasons, it is impossible to work and this must be acknowledged.

Whatever the reason for your decision, you must be careful when expressing your assessment to be clear and nurturing to the patient. Do not attach blame or destroy hope, and be as positive as the condition or situation will allow. Where relevant you may refer the patient to a more experienced practitioner in your own field, or to a different therapy. Do not withdraw the potential for support while it may still be needed.

How do I keep my knowledge up to date?

This is obviously an ongoing process. You will need to subscribe to professional journals, including the Association of Natural Medicine (ANM) quarterly journal - 'Natural Medicine', and to read them regularly. The Practitioner Days which are offered by the ANM give a broad spread of lectures and further training.

If you are aware of any weak areas in your knowledge, it is your responsibility as a practitioner to read further, investigate, visit libraries, contact other practitioners, or seek further training.

You are requested to attend a minimum of two days on-going professional training/development annually and to supply evidence of this when re-applying for membership.

Your initial training course is often the beginning of a fascinating and stimulating journey of discovery. We need never stop learning! The ANM requires of its Registered Members Continuing Professional Development (CPD).

CPD is an on-going lifelong process of learning from the point of your initial/basic qualification regarding your chosen therapy/ies. CPD facilitates your progress and growth as a practitioner and helps maintain your own and your profession's credibility and identity. CPD requires from you an investment in how you are ensuring you meet the care needs and interests of your patients in the best professional way possible.

(See *How can I evaluate my work?*)

How can I evaluate my work?

There are various approaches to evaluating the quality of your work. The maintenance of standards being of central consideration. You can: (Knight 1992)

- Look at the entire process with given individual patients to answer effectiveness, strengths and weaknesses in the process.

- You can select particular points in the process, for example case taking, for closer scrutiny.

- Evaluate the quality of your interaction with the patient.

- You can work in conjunction with the patient, review process and ask for feedback.

- You can ask for supervision from a neutral party.

Self evaluation for the effective practitioner is an integral aspect of the total helping process. This ongoing evaluation provides the information upon which your further development and acquisition of skill can be planned and guided. Of course, underlying any meaningful self evaluation must be your own motivation to enrich and promote your own abilities.

Supervision and peer group support with the opportunity to relate academic learning and your own developing experience is invaluable. Moreover the involvement of patients directly in evaluating your practice is to be recommended. It is a question of evaluating your practice and then relating findings to your overall professional development as well as your future learning requirements.

The success of the helping relationship depends on the performance of the practitioner - how well you, the practitioner, use your intuitions, your training and how well you are able to relate to the patient. Practitioners are in a difficult position in that they aim to encourage patients of widely different abilities, insights and motivation to 'perform' to the best of their ability. Clearly practitioners familiar with principles of individual differences and their implications for the helping process may also need to be ingenious in vitalising some patients in terms of confidence and security. Your competence is fundamental to any consideration of effectiveness in fulfilling the helping task and in doing so will take the responsibility for:

- Observing the Code of Ethics.

- Informing the patient of methods and principles to be used as well as the duration of sessions and fees (if any).

- Exploring with the patient their own expectations of what is involved in their treatment.

- Confirming with the patient whether or not they are currently involved in any other therapy and if yes, and if appropriate, gaining the patient's permission before conferring with other professsionals.

- Taking account of your own competence and making referral when necessary.

- Terminating treatment when the patient has received the help sought or when it is apparent that your 'help' is no longer helping.

- Increasing your own professional development and also monitoring the limits of your competence.

- Being actively involved in developing your own wholeness.

- Approaching from a position of humility with the understanding that each of us has needs - the person being helped and the person helping.

- Recognising that the patient also has strengths and being aware of this fact.

Who looks after me the practitioner?

Ultimately the responsibility lies with you, but there is support available. The Association of Natural Medicine will be happy to refer you to a professional if you need to discuss a case, or indeed any personal problems, in total confidentiality. You are strongly advised to arrange regular personal supervision sessions, where you can raise issues which concern you, offload some of the pain you may have absorbed and feel nurtured by having time to focus on your professional work.

Often it helps to follow your own advice to patients - for example to eat well, rest, recharge, play, and monitor stress levels. If you do not look after yourself you will be unable to offer the best treatment to your patients.

The ANM runs regular practitioner support days, seminars and professional development workshops. Make sure you attend as many as you can.

ANNEX 1
Association of Natural Medicine Disciplinary Procedure

1. GENERAL GUIDANCE

1.1 The scope of the following Disciplinary Procedure relates to all Registered Members of the Association of Natural Medicines (RMANM) and qualified Members of the Association of Natural Medicine (MANM).

1.2 The Procedure takes due account of the ANM Code of Ethics and the expectation that all RM/MANM adhere fully to that Code of Ethics and the professional standards embraced therein.

1.3 Where the standard of practice of a RM/MANM is below the standards set within the Code of Ethics then this will normally be dealt with as a case of professional misconduct and become subject to the ANM Disciplinary Procedure.

1.4 The ANM is concerned that all of its RM/MANM should be aware of their obligations with regard to conduct including standards of professional practice and of the likely consequences of the failure to meet these obligations as indicated by this Disciplinary Procedure.

1.5 The ANM accepts that it has an obligation to ensure, so far as is reasonably practical, that all RM/MANM are appropriately qualified to practise their particular specialism/s prior to Registration.

1.6 The ANM assumes responsibility for ensuring that the Code of Ethics is made available to all RM/MANM.

1.7 The ANM also assumes that all RM/MANM have the responsibility to familiarise themselves with the Code of Ethics and such amendments as may be made and drawn to their attention from time to time.

1.8 The ANM will maintain and make available on request to any member of the public a list of RM/MANM, the Code of Ethics, and Disciplinary Procedure.

2. THE INVESTIGATION

2.1 Where a RM/MANM conduct or standard of performance is called into question, a member of the Governing Council (GC) shall conduct, or cause to be conducted, such investigation as he/she may consider necessary including, where appropriate, giving the Registered Member ample opportunity to state his/her case. If, in consequence, the member of the GC considers formal disciplinary action on the matter needs to follow he/she shall arrange for a disciplinary hearing accordingly.

2.2 When determining disciplinary action to be taken, the need must be born in mind of satisfying the test of reasonableness in all the circumstances. Account should be taken of the RM/MANM record and any other relevant factors.

2.3 Formal Disciplinary Action will not be taken against a RM/MANM without prior investigation.

2.4 Where the member of the GC forms the view that, in a case which is apparently of gross or serious misconduct, the circumstances require the suspension of the RM/MANM pending the Disciplinary Hearing, he/she shall advise the Chief Executive/President of the ANM who may suspend the RM/MANM and shall inform the GC of the action taken.

2.5 Alleged gross misconduct will normally lead to immediate suspension of a RM/MANM pending a disciplinary hearing and, if confirmed at the disciplinary hearing, will result in summary removal from the ANM Register.

2.6 If at the Disciplinary Hearing the allegations are not confirmed then the RM/MANM will be reinstated and suspension cease.

NOTE

The following list provides examples, which will be considered as gross or serious misconduct:

* The deliberate falsification of qualifications.

* Assault on another person.

* Serious incapability through alcohol or being under the influence of illegal drugs.

3.   DISCIPLINARY HEARING: PRINCIPLES

3.1   No disciplinary action will be taken against a RM/MANM until the case has been fully investigated by a member of the Governing Council.

3.2   At every stage of the Procedure the RM/MANM will be advised of the nature of the complaint against him or her and will be given the opportunity to state his/her case before any decision is made.

3.3   At all stages the RM/MANM will have the right to be accompanied by a representative or colleague during the Disciplinary Hearing.

3.4   No RM/MANM will be deregistered for a first breach of discipline, except in the case of gross misconduct.

3.5   A RM/MANM will have no right of appeal against any decision reached at the hearing.

4.   THE PROCEDURE

4.1   The procedure is designed to establish the facts quickly and to deal consistently with disciplinary issues. No disciplinary action will be taken until the matter has been fully investigated.

4.2   At every stage the RM/MANM will have the opportunity to state their case and be represented, if they wish, at the Disciplinary Hearing.

4.3   A RM/MANM has no right to appeal against any disciplinary penalty.

4.4   The RM/MANM will be given notice in writing at least 15 days in advance of the hearing.

4.5   The Disciplinary Panel hearing the disciplinary matter will consist of a minimum of two members of the ANM GC and will be chaired by an independent person drawn from the ANM Charity sub-committee.

4.6   The ANM representative, the member of the Governing Council who conducted the investigation, will put the case in the presence of the RM/MANM and his representative and may call witnesses.

4.7   The RM/MANM and/or his/her representative will have the opportunity to ask questions of the ANM representative on the evidence given by him and any witnesses whom he may call and on any relevant aspect of the case.

4.8   The RM/MANM will put his case in the presence of the ANM representative.

4.9   The ANM Disciplinary Panel will deliberate in private and may recall the RM/MANM and/or his/her representative to clear points of uncertainty on evidence already given.

4.10 The ANM Disciplinary Panel will announce the decision to the RM/ MANM or his/her representative personally or in writing, as they may determine.

5. DISCIPLINARY RECORDS

5.1 Any records relating to disciplinary proceedings will be carefully safeguarded and kept strictly confidential. Should any disciplinary action in the event be found to be unwarranted, any written reference thereto will be removed from the ANM records.

6. GUIDANCE AS TO ACTION WHICH MAY BE TAKEN BY THE ANM DISCIPLINARY PANEL

6.1 Minor faults will be dealt with informally, but where the matter is more serious the following guidance will be used.

6.2 Oral warning:
If conduct or performance does not meet acceptable standards, the RM/MANM will normally be given a formal oral warning. He/she will be advised of the reason for the warning. A brief note of the oral warning will be kept but it will be spent after twelve months subject to satisfactory conduct and performance.

6.3   Written warning:

If the offence is a serious one, or if a further offence occurs, a written warning will be given to the RM/MANM by the President of the ANM. This will give details of the complaint, the improvement required and the time scale. It will warn that further action under this Disciplinary Procedure will be considered if there is no satisfactory improvement. A copy of this written warning will be kept by the ANM and will be disregarded for disciplinary purposes after twelve months subject to satisfactory conduct and performance.

6.4   If there is still a failure to improve, or conduct or performance is still unsatisfactory, or if the RM/MANM fails to reach the prescribed standards, de-registration will normally result.

ANNEX 2
Application for Training or Registration as a Member of the Association of Natural Medicine (ANM)

1. It is the policy of the ANM to require all applicants for training or Registration as a Member of the ANM to disclose criminal convictions.

2. The Rehabilitation of Offenders Act 1974 provides that certain convictions shall be regarded as 'spent' after specified periods of time have elapsed and you do not need to disclose convictions which are 'spent' at the date you sign the application form. You are, however, required to disclose all 'unspent' criminal convictions.

3. Please remember that a conviction includes:
    a) A sentence of imprisonment, youth custody or borstal training.
    b) An absolute discharge, conditional discharge, bind over.
    c) A fit person order, a supervision or care order, a probation order or an approved school order arising from a criminal conviction.
    d) Simple dismissal from the Armed Forces, cashiering, discharge with ignominy, dismissal with disgrace or detention by the Armed Forces.
    e) Detention by direction of the Home Secretary
    f) Detention centre, remand home, or attendance centre orders.
    g) A suspended sentence

h) A fine or any other sentence not mentioned above.

4.   I confirm the following convictions -

5.   Or
I certify that I have no convictions to declare and I understand that any false information could lead to disciplinary action by the ANM.

Name...(please use capitals)

Signature...

Date................................

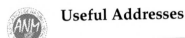

Association of Natural Medicine
19a Collingwood Road, Witham, Essex CM8 2DY
Telephone/Fax   01376 502762
Website   www.associationnaturalmedicine.co.uk

Business Link for Essex
Alexandra House, 36a Church Street, Gt Beddow, Chelmsford CM2 7HY
Telephone   01245 241400
Fax   01245 241500
Email   info@BL4E.co.uk

Chelmsford Enterprise Agency
Unit 3, Robjohns House, Navigation Road, Chelmsford, Essex CM2 6ND
Telephone   01245 496712

Data Protection Registrar
Wycliffe House, Water Lane, Wilmslow, Cheshire SK9 5AF

Department of Trade and Industry - Eastern Area Office, Building A, Westbrooks Research Centre, Milton Road, Cambridge CB4 1YG

Dr Edward Bach Centre
Mount Vernon, Sotwell, Wallingford, Oxen OX10 0PZ
Telephone   01491 834678
Email   mail@bachcentre.com
Website   www.bachcentre.com

Guidance on Data Protection
Office of the Information Commissioner, Wycliffe
House, Water Lane, Wilmslow, Cheshire SK9 5AF
Information line   01625 545745
Notification line   01635 545740
Website   www.dataprotection.gov.uk

HSE Books *(for free publications about Health and Safety)*
PO Box 1999, Sudbury, Suffolk CO10 2WA
Telephone   01787 881165
Fax   01787 313995
Website   www.hsebooks.co.uk

Institute of Chartered Accountants
PO Box 433, Chartered Accountants Hall, Moorgate
Place, London
EC2P 2BJ

Mr Jack Lawrence *(for Insurance advice)*
1 Orchard Villas, Colebrook, Plymouth, Devon PL7 4EZ
Telephone   01752 340740

Medicine-Healthcare Products
Regulating Agency, Market Towers, 1 Nine Elms Lane,
London SW8 5NQ
Telephone   020 7084 2000
Website   www.europa.eu.int

Practitioners wishing to work abroad should contact
the British Embassy regarding the legalities of working
in any given country.

Bibliography

Autton N   Touch, An Exploration. Darton. Long-
                    man & Todd Ltd, 1984

Compton B R   Social Work Processes, Dorsey, 1975
& Galaway B

Farrah D   The Nurse, The Patient + Touch in Cur-
                    rent Concepts in Clinical Nursing, Eds
                    M Dutley, E M Anderson, B S Berger-
                    son, M Lohr & M H Rose. The C V
                    Mosdy Co, Lt Louis, 1971

Jacoby M   'The Analytic Encounter' Inner City
                    Books, 1982

Jamieson J   'What is an interview' Community
                    Care No.1998, 1978

Knight R A   'Let Me Tell You Who I Am', Cross
                    Roads Publications, 1992 (Available
                    from the Association of Natural Medi-
                    cine)

Menninger K   Theory of Psychoardytic Tech, Basic
                    Books, New York,1958

Older J   Touching is Healing, Stein & Day Pub,
                    New York, 1982

Patterson J E   Effects of Touch on self exploration and the therapeutic relationship, Counselling & Clinical Psychology, 1975

Rogers C R   'The Therapeutic Relationship and its Impact', University of Wisconsin Press, 1967

Wolberg S   The Technique of Psychotherapy, Grune + Stratton, New York, 1954

Index

The Authors

Richard Knight graduated both from London and Birmingham Universities and holds professional qualifications in social work, education and philosophy. He researched Transactional Analysis at the Cathexis Institute in California and completed the Senior Course in Criminology at Cambridge University. Richard has lectured and run workshops Nationally on the management and treatment of disturbed children for Central Government Departments and other organisations. For the past thirty-six years he has worked in the helping profession, was responsible for developing the counselling module in the Association of Natural Medicine training course, is a member of their Governing Council and also a Fellow of the Royal Society of Arts. His Doctorate is in Psychotherapy and Counselling.

Bridget Main is a qualified homeopath specialising in allergies and has been running her own practice for over six years. Her work is influenced by the yogic tradition and she has been a qualified teacher through the British Wheel of Yoga since 1978.

In addition to running her clinic she has undertaken advanced training in homeopathy in India, and was the company secretary to the ANM for fifteen years.

Janet Robinson qualified with the ANM in homeopathy, counselling and naturopathy and is a British Wheel of Yoga teacher.

In 1992 Janet completed post graduate advanced study as a Homoeopathic Physician at the Bengal Allen Medical Institute which in addition to clinical experience in hospital also involved working with the poor in the community. Janet practices homeopathy at her own clinic in Earls Colne, Essex and teaches classical homeopathy.

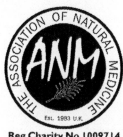